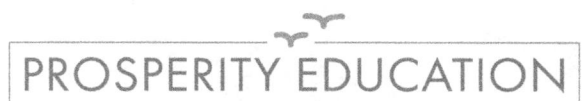

OET Reading

Six practice tests for the Occupational English Test

Alecia Banfield

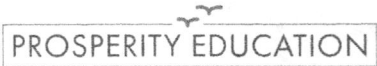

© Prosperity Education Ltd. 2025

Registered offices: Sherlock Close, Cambridge
CB3 0HP, United Kingdom

First published 2025

ISBN: 978-1-915654-21-2

This publication is in copyright. Subject to statutory exception and to the provisions of relevant collective licensing agreements, no reproduction of any part may take place without the written permission of Prosperity Education.

The moral right of the author has been asserted.

'OET' is a brand belonging to the Cambridge Boxhill Language Assessment Trust (CBLA), and is not associated with Prosperity Education or its products.

Designed by ORP Cambridge

For further information and resources, visit:
www.prosperityeducation.net

To infinity and beyond.

Contents

Introduction to the OET Reading subtest   *v*

Test 1   *1*

Test 2   *23*

Test 3   *45*

Test 4   *67*

Test 5   *89*

Test 6   *111*

Answers   *133*

Dr. Alecia Banfield (MBBS, MPH, TEFL/TESOL) is a Medical English specialist and a certified OET Premium Preparation Partner who has helped thousands of healthcare professionals achieve exam success.

Introduction to the OET Reading subtest

The Occupational English Test (OET) assesses professional language communication skills specifically within the high-stake contexts of clinical and non-clinical healthcare. It is accepted by governments and immigration authorities as evidence of advanced English comprehension and production, and it is currently available for 12 professions: Dentistry, Dietetics, Medicine, Nursing, Occupational Therapy, Optometry, Pharmacy, Physiotherapy, Podiatry, Radiography, Speech Pathology and Veterinary Science. Candidates may take either a paper- or computer-based test, and this choice can impact aspects of their preparation.

The test itself consists of four subtests: Listening, Reading, Writing and Speaking, and candidates must pass all four subtests to be considered successful. This ensures that OET candidates are genuinely able to comprehend and produce English independently, competently and appropriately within the full range of standard, on-the-job communication modalities. All professions take the same Reading and Listening subtests, while the Writing and Speaking subtests are profession-specific.

This book focuses solely on Reading, providing six standardised, complete Reading practice tests appropriate for teachers and candidates alike.

The OET Reading subtest

The Reading subtest lasts for 60 minutes and is divided into three parts:

Part A
- 4 short texts (A, B, C and D) of the types encountered in direct patient care, e.g. disease-reference information, diagnostic algorithms, treatment regimens and approaches to known complications. They may be presented as paragraphs, bullet points, flow charts, tables or graphs.
- 20 short-answer questions based on the texts.
- Completion time: 15 minutes.

On completion of Part A, access to the paper ends and there is no further opportunity to review or amend answers.

Part B
- 6 questions, each with a short text of 100–150 words concerning non-clinical activities, e.g. device instructions, administrative procedures, staff protocols and advisories, and institution policies.
- Each multiple-choice question has 3 answer options.

Part C
- Two texts of 800–900 words, each divided into 7–8 paragraphs. They feature non-clinical information typical of, e.g. research, professional editorials and opinions, and other continuing professional education content.
- Each text has 8 multiple-choice questions with 4 answer options to choose from.

Parts B and C are presented together and last 45 minutes in total.

Challenges of the OET Reading subtest

The different kinds of content and layout, together with the time pressure, require candidates to not only be confident in their control of language but also proficiently display a range of strategies and skills for each part.

Reading Part A

The 20 questions in this part are divided into three sections:

Questions 1–7   Use letters A, B, C and D only to identify where information is found.

Example:
Text A – *the typical features of disease X.*
Text B – *tests that confirm or rule out disease X.*
Text C – *a specific complication of X.*
Text D – *steps in a technical procedure related to X.*

Question: *Where would you find symptoms that suggest a patient does not have disease X?*

Answer: *B.*

Skills needed: Fast reading comprehension and ability to deploy a wide vocabulary for rephrasing; understanding the different ways in which content can be presented and how it logically flows. The candidate should know that 'rule out" and 'suggest the patient does not have' mean the same thing. However, quickly skimming the text headings may suggest more than one text to be a possible answer (e.g. also Text A). For this reason, the candidate should also quickly scan within other possible texts to confirm the location of the information. They should not choose based only on the text heading.

Questions 8–14   Give a short 1–3-word answer to a question, exactly as it appears in the text.

Example:
Text C: *If complications occur, start drug Y at 10 mg/kg and increase until the patient stabilises. Do not exceed 20mg/kg.*

Question: *What is the maximum dose of drug Y that can be given?*

Answer: *20mg/kg.*

Skills needed: Wide vocabulary to identify that 'maximum dose' and 'do not exceed' mean the same thing; fast reading skills to find the right text and right information; and precise copying. Note that, in haste, a candidate may write only '20mg'. This would be wrong as '20 mg' is the maximum dose *per kg* and not *the maximum total dose.* It is important to pay close attention to what actually is being asked.

Questions 15–20   Complete a sentence with a short 1-3-word answer exactly as it appears in a text.

Example:
Text D: *Review site at regular intervals, especially for the beginning of suppuration.*

Question: *It is important to check sites frequently to detect early _____.*

Answer: *suppuration*

Skills needed: Wide vocabulary to identify 'beginning of' as meaning 'early'; fast reading skills to find the right text and right information; and precise copying. Even if a candidate does not know the word 'suppuration', they should copy the spelling correctly. Candidates should be comfortable encountering occasional new words without this distracting them or unduly affecting their confidence.

Reading Part B

This part tests deeper and broader meaning of language as opposed to spelling, vocabulary and grammar. Candidates should understand the main point or the gist of a text, and be able to recognise purpose of communication, action-and-consequence relationships, inference and rephrasing.

Example:
- Text: *Staff should know their recertification deadline and complete recertification before the end of their previous cycle. Failure to hold recertification credentials for any duration of time can result in temporary or permanent interruption of employment status.*
- Answer: (Inference; rephrasing) *An employee could be fired if their previous certification expires before they recertify.*

Reading Part C

This can prove the most challenging part of the subtest due to the length of the two texts, the advanced language used and four answer options to choose from instead of three.

For this reason, in preparation, candidates should purposely practise increasing their 'reading stamina' – that is, practise focusing on the meaning of increasingly longer texts until reading and understanding for a continuous 60 minutes is no longer a challenge.

Other language skills tested include understanding a text's main point, purpose and call to action for the reader, as well as gist, action and consequence, inference, rephrasing, the grammar of substitution and deducing the meaning of idioms based on context or the language around them. Again, candidates will very likely encounter a term that is new, but this should not completely hinder their comprehension of the rest of information around it.

All these skills are covered in the design of these original, standardised Reading practice tests. I hope that teachers and candidates find this a useful resource in identifying and strengthening areas for language improvement while reinforcing areas in which candidates are justified in being confident.

Dr. Alecia Banfield (MBBS, MPH, TEFL/TESOL)

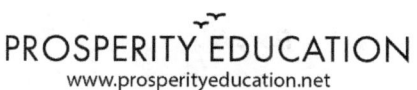

Occupational English Test

Reading

Test 1

© 2025 Prosperity Education
'OET' is a brand belonging to the Cambridge Boxhill Language Assessment Trust (CBLA),
and is not associated with Prosperity Education or its products.

Part A

- Look at the four texts (**A–D**) in the accompanying **text booklet**.
- For each question (**1–20**) look through the texts (**A–D**) to find the relevant information.
- Write your answers in the spaces provided in this **question paper**.
- Answer all the questions within the 15-minute time limit.
- Your answers should **only** be taken from texts **A–D** and must be correctly spelt.

Smoking and Nicotine: Questions

Questions 1–7

For each question (**1–7**), decide which text (**A, B, C** or **D**) the information comes from. Write the letter **A, B, C** or **D** in the space provided. You may use any letter more than once.

In which text can you find information about

1. comparisons between toxins in regular cigarettes and e-cigarettes? _____

2. how too much nicotine can be absorbed into a person's body? _____

3. how pharmaceutical therapies work? _____

4. sensations smokers might experience when they first stop smoking? _____

5. a specific behaviour those trying to reduce smoking tend to engage in? _____

6. how the cardiovascular system reacts when nicotine enters the body? _____

7. what happens if persons develop mental disorders while on certain drugs? _____

Questions 8–14

Answer each of the questions (**8–14**) with a word or short phrase from one of the texts. Each answer may include words, numbers or both. You should **not** write full sentences.

8. Which medication is very effective on its own in treating nicotine-withdrawal symptoms?

    _____

9. How long can someone expect to feel ill if small amounts of pure nicotine enter their body?

    _____

Test 1 | Part A

10 What is the maximum time it takes for nicotine to enter the body and reach the brain?

_____

11 What symptom does the majority of people with nicotine poisoning have?

_____

12 What should the practitioner organise at each visit to help the patient not restart smoking?

_____

13 What should a smoker have at the same time they are receiving pharmaceutical therapy?

_____

14 What is the minimum time that must lapse between finishing MAOI drugs and starting bupropion?

_____

Questions 15–20

Complete each of the sentences (15–20) with a word or short phrase from one of the texts. Each answer may include words, numbers or both.

15 During pregnancy, a smoker is at increased risk of _____.

16 Some cessation drugs work by preventing the brain from registering _____ when nicotine is consumed.

17 When helping smokers to quit, qualified practitioners should use interventions that are _____.

18 Sleep disturbance can occur in as few as _____ after quitting smoking.

19 After 30 minutes, cardiovascular signs shown in nicotine poisoning include irregular heartbeat, low blood pressure and _____.

20 Nicotine-replacement patches are contraindicated in persons who have inflamed or _____ skin.

End of Part A

Smoking and Nicotine: Texts

Text A

General Guidance for Professionals

Smoking is a chronic disorder and the optimal approach used by licensed professionals for helping smokers to cease should be in keeping with guidelines for any chronic-disease management: continually assessing and monitoring status, using evidence-based interventions and encouraging abstinence from or reduction in harmful behaviours. However, smokers should be made aware that people who only reduce the number of cigarettes they smoke tend to compensate by inhaling more of the smoke each time in order to maintain the nicotine intake, and so may not actually improve their health in comparison to those who stop smoking completely.

Conversations with someone who declares a desire to quit smoking should review smoking history, the smoking habits of close acquaintances and previous cessation attempts. For those who opt for tapering their daily cigarette count, a 'complete stop' date should be agreed.

Counselling at each appointment should include: emphasising the benefits of stopping tobacco use, encouraging the use of evidence-based medications and combination therapies and arranging timely follow-up appointments to help stave off relapse.

Text B

Specific Advice to Give Smokers

General Health: Harmful chemicals in cigarettes have been shown to cause

- cancer
- heart and lung disease
- diabetes
- osteoporosis, rheumatoid arthritis
- cataracts
- male erectile dysfunction

Maternal and Baby Issues:

- decreased fertility; increased miscarriage risk
- low birth weight
- sudden infant death syndrome (SIDS)

Dangers of Nicotine:

- Addiction: nicotine travels directly across the mucous lining of the mouth and lungs to the blood then to the brain in eight-to-ten seconds. There, it triggers natural chemicals such as dopamine.

- Withdrawal: withdrawal symptoms can start within one-to-three days of stopping, and include: cough, headaches, constipation, anxiety/depression, inability to concentrate, irritability, insomnia, hunger, headaches, gastrointestinal disturbances and insomnia.

- Cigarette cravings can continue for years.

Emphasise that a wide range of therapies is available, and that most therapies are best used in combination.

Text C

Risk of Nicotine Toxicity with E-cigarettes

There are fewer pollutants in e-cigarettes, but their liquid-nicotine content can increase the risk of addiction and toxicity beyond that of normal cigarettes.

Some e-cigarette devices can deliver 5000-to-6000 puffs from one filling, which is the equivalent of 500-to-600 cigarettes or 25-to-30 packs of cigarettes. This can place users at risk of nicotine poisoning if their e-cigarette use is excessive.

Nicotine overdose can also occur from direct contact with insecticides containing nicotine. A lethal dose of inhaled nicotine is 50-to-60 mg/kg in a 70-kg adult.

Symptoms and Signs

Early phase (<15 minutes after nicotine enters the body):

- Vomiting (in >50% of cases)
- Increased salivation
- Abdominal pain
- Sweating and pallor
- Increased blood pressure and pulse rate
- Rapid, heavy breathing (hyperpnea)
- Twitching, ataxia and loss of balance
- Headache; dizziness

Late phase:

- Diarrhoea
- Arrhythmias, hypotension and bradycardia
- Muscle weakness/paralysis
- Shallow breathing; respiratory failure
- Coma

Duration

- Mild exposure: 1–2 hours
- Severe exposure: 18–24 hours. Death can occur.

Poisoning is more common in children due to their smaller body size. Symptoms include: vomiting, rapid heart rate, unsteadiness and increased salivation.

Text D

Adult Drug Therapies

Combinations of different drug therapies tend to be more effective than single products, although varenicline demonstrates high efficacy as monotherapy. For best results, a long-acting nicotine-replacement therapy (e.g. nicotine patches) should be combined with a shorter-acting form (e.g. gum or spray).

Drugs should also be taken simultaneously in conjunction with cognitive behavioural counseling.

Contraindications: pregnancy; <18 years old; use of smokeless tobacco

Medication	Mechanism of Action	Administration	Cautions
Bupropion SR	Increases the brain's release of norepinephrine and dopamine.	150mg oral, once daily After 3 days 150mg oral, twice daily After several weeks 200mg oral, twice daily Max. 400mg/day Used for 7–12 weeks, and up to 6 months	Contraindicated in seizures, eating disorders, and monoamine oxidase inhibitors taken within the previous two weeks (may cause *neuropsychiatric effects).
Varenicline (monotherapy) Nasal spray, oral tabs	Binds and blocks nicotine receptors, preventing the brain from feeling pleasure. Also has some effects similar to nicotine but does not trigger withdrawal when drug is stopped.	0.5mg oral, once daily After 3 days 0.5mg oral, twice daily After 7 days 1mg oral, twice daily Used for 12–24 weeks. Better long-term abstinence with use of >12 weeks	Can cause nausea, sleep disturbance, and also *neuropsychiatric effects.
Nicotine-replacement therapies (gum, lozenge, nasal spray, patch)	Alternative source of nicotine delivered to brain at lower rate to reduce risk of addiction.	1mg of nicotine replacement per cigarette smoked per day Gum and lozenges used for up to 6 months Nasal spray used for 14 weeks Patch used for 10 weeks	Careful use in diabetes, hyperthyroidism, and high-risk cardiovascular disease (e.g. recent heart attack or arrythmia). Patches contraindicated in skin inflammation or sensitivity. Patch use should continue even if patients lapse and smoke. Nasal spray can cause nasopharyngeal irritation.

*Immediate cessation of drug indicated. Patients should be monitored until any depression, aggression and/or suicidal thoughts abate completely.

End of Part A | Text booklet

Part B

In this part of the test, there are six short extracts relating to the work of health professionals. For questions **1–6**, choose the answer (**A**, **B** or **C**) that you think fits best according to the text.

Your answers should be made by filling in the circle completely: Ⓐ ● Ⓒ

1. The guidelines suggest that

   Ⓐ staff without specialty bariatric training should not be involved in moving obese patients.

   Ⓑ two staff members are needed to manoeuvre a patient if using a ceiling-lift device.

   Ⓒ if there is no specialty bariatric suite available, an elective admission cannot occur.

Guidelines – Elective Admission Of Obese (Bariatric) Patients

Bariatric patients (BMI >40) require more frequent repositioning than normal-weighted patients to prevent pressure ulcers and respiratory issues, and to assist wound healing. Both they and attending staff are at increased risk of traumatic injury during bed transfers, repositioning and bathroom activities. Therefore, safety in handling bariatric patients should start before admission, with staff training and a review of rooms and required equipment. Patient-specific and staffing needs should also be documented.

If a bariatric suite is not available, a regular room should be identified for adaptation, allowing space for patient, equipment and manoeuvring. How many people are required to operate each piece of equipment safely should be mapped out. It is against guidelines for any staff member to move a bariatric patient alone, whether or not the staff member has received specific training or specialised equipment is being used. Three staff members are required to safely move a patient into and out of bed using a mobile floor lift, while operation of the attached ceiling lifts requires fewer persons.

There is sometimes the perception that specialty equipment is inconvenient to use or difficult to locate, especially when under time constraints, and staff resort to unsafe practices as a consequence. Relying solely on body mechanics to mobilise bariatric patients is ill-advised.

2. The guidelines suggest that

   (A) the admitting physician is not automatically qualified to verify patient EIP self-management.

   (B) the patient is not required to sign the EIP self-management consent form.

   (C) taking any kind of drug disqualifies a person from managing an EIP.

In-Patient External Insulin Pumps

If a physician is admitting a diabetic patient who is using an external insulin pump (EIP), it must be determined whether the pump can remain in place, and whether the patient or a responsible accompanying adult guardian is capable of managing it correctly throughout the patient's hospital stay. These points must be verified within the first 12 hours by either an endocrinologist, hospital diabetes management service or physician specially trained in EIP management. The person managing the EIP must sign a consent form outlining their responsibilities.

Consider the following to determine whether the patient or the accompanying adult guardian is capable of monitoring the EIP:

- Is the person managing the pump alert, knowledgeable, physically capable and, in the case of the adult guardian, available 24 hours a day and 7 days a week?
- Does the person managing the EIP demonstrate knowledge of hypoglycaemia symptoms?
- Are they able to calculate and administer bolus doses via the pump, stop insulin delivery and adjust infusion rates?
- Are they willing to provide the required pump supplies?

Contraindications to managing the EIP include altered alertness (e.g. being under the influence of illicit drugs), being disorientated or showing any physical or mental problem.

3. The main purpose of the instructions is to

   (A) raise awareness of the kind of harm some discarded drugs pose if discarded incorrectly.

   (B) identify which drugs can go into household waste and which need special considerations.

   (C) send a warning about unused or expired drugs that can harm the environment.

Advisory – Disposal of Unused or Expired Drugs
Unused or expired drugs should ideally be returned to a drug take-back facility. However, this may not always be available or feasible. Other options for disposing of medications depend on the class of drug. Drugs listed on the 'flush list' should be flushed down the toilet as they have been classed as having misuse- or abuse-potential and/or carry a higher chance of causing death if a single dose is taken other than as prescribed. Such drugs can pose a danger to children, adults or pets if accidentally or intentionally ingested or touched. For other medicines, follow the individual guidelines for discarding, including with domestic waste. The relevant authorities and pharmaceutical manufacturers are aware of the debate surrounding what potential harm discarded medicines pose to the environment. The above guidelines have been developed after weighing the risks against the benefits.

4. The memo states that

   (A) the care home must legally have an exercise programme.

   (B) patients who qualify for the programme will participate twice weekly.

   (C) the programme will reduce the risks to patients.

TO: Residential Care Staff

TOPIC: "Get Moving" Exercise Programme for the Elderly

Next month will be the launch of our fitness programme for elderly residents. Participation in this voluntary programme will be based on mobility, cognitive function, medical aid use and previous history of falls.

Residential care homes have a legal obligation to reduce or prevent falls, and muscle weakness and poor gait contribute to a quarter of falls in nursing homes in this country. While there are no national guidelines for residential care fitness programmes, WHO 2020 recommends those ≥65 years have 150–300 minutes of moderate exercise or 75–150 min of vigorous exercise weekly. Supervised combination training has been shown to be safe, prevent falls, to slow physical and cognitive decline and improve quality of life.

'Get Moving' includes aerobic, balance, flexibility training and strength training, and will be supervised by qualified personnel.

All residents meeting the participation criteria should be strongly encouraged to participate at least twice per week.

5. The main purpose of the text is to

   (A) explain the EHS regulations that eyewash-station inspectors follow.

   (B) help users recognise when a station is safe to use.

   (C) give guidelines on the correct maintenance schedule for eyewash stations.

Emergency Eyewash Stations
Eyewash stations must be maintained and flushed once a week, in accordance with Environmental Health and Safety (EHS) inspection requirements. Weekly flushes prevent stagnant bacteria, dust and rust particles from accumulating between cap and spray-head or in the irrigation line, potentially harming users' eyes in an emergency.
A well-designed and functioning eyewash station should have a clear, lukewarm stream of water that projects upwards at a pressure that allows the user to use it comfortably for 15 minutes continuously.
There should be a conveniently placed gripping handle for stability, and it should not be obstructed by other objects such as towels and rags. The interface between the spray-head and the cap should be cleaned with 70% ethanol or isopropanol.
Conducting inspections during regular working hours increases the likelihood of detecting problems that might otherwise go unnoticed.

6. Guidelines in the text suggests that

   (A) persons not related to the dementia patient can play a role in determining whether or not the patient can give their own consent.

   (B) healthcare staff should first follow legal guidelines in deciding whether to accept consent for care from a dementia patient.

   (C) an MMSE must be conducted more than once before a patient with dementia is allowed to sign their own consent form.

Guidelines – Consent In Dementia Patients

Having dementia does not mean that a person cannot give consent to their own care. A mental-capacity assessment or mini mental-status examination (MMSE) should be conducted (more than once, if indicated) before a finding is made. Even then, a MMSE score on its own cannot be taken as sufficient proof of capabilities until and unless all practicable steps to assist the patient have been taken.

Carers play an important role as they can potentially share longstanding knowledge of the patient's cognitive functioning. Information should be given to the patient in writing, preferably in the presence of an adult listed as their next of kin or emergency contact. The patient should have ample opportunity to read and ask questions about this information, and they should be invited to repeat the discussion at another time if their cognitive function is known to fluctuate. Any consent the patient then gives should also be in writing.

Where dementia patients do not have capacity to consent and there is no contact person or next of kin available, healthcare staff must act in the best interests of the patient, and also bear in mind the Mental Health Act and medico-legal regulations.

End of Part B

Part C

In this part of the test, there are two texts about different aspects of healthcare. For questions **7–22**, choose the answer (**A**, **B**, **C** or **D**) that you think fits best according to the text.

Your answers should be made by filling in the circle completely: Ⓐ Ⓑ Ⓒ Ⓓ

Text 1: Clinician Grief

Grief is an intensely personal yet universal state and process. Between the 1940s and 1990s, research into grief focused on key terms relevant to specific social groups or events such as the aged and stillbirths, and within communities most affected by the AIDS epidemic. Since then, there has been increasing investigation into how we process grief, with key terms that include chronic stress, bereavement-related depression, death and palliative care. In the wake of the COVID-19 pandemic, there has been a further surge of interest in aspects such as the complexities and challenges of grief and its impact on mental well-being.

Features of grief include shock, sadness, anger and guilt, and a loss of interest in things previously enjoyed. There can even be physical symptoms such as fatigue, nausea and headaches. Researchers now define normal grief and also complicated grief that might develop in sudden and unexpected loss. *The Diagnostic and Statistical Manual 5* further describes prolonged grief disorder (PGD), post-traumatic stress disorder (PTSD) and clinical depression. These classifications can help in the identification of those needing professional intervention. Many factors contribute to complicating grief. Disenfranchised grief, for instance, occurs when the person cannot openly mourn, or it can be complicated when they are left with unresolved issues concerning the person who has died. In fact, it has been found that the pre-death experiences with the dying person are as important as, if not more important than, what is done to help the bereaved person after the death has occurred. This led researchers, S.E. Morris and S.D. Block, to suggest that bereavement care and counseling are best tackled as a 'preventive model'.

Healthcare professionals (HCP) not only experience natural losses in their personal lives, but also many losses in their professional lives. A patient's death may feel like a personal loss, or there may be anger about missed opportunities to prevent a death. It is heartening, therefore, that some healthcare professions explicitly confront their own grief in integrated training. For oncology and palliative care nurses, an outstanding programme called 'Songs for the Soul' combines the healing effects of expressive writing, storytelling and music to help nurses. Physician education, however, measures success in terms of conquering disease and pushing back death. This mindset runs counter to accepting death and exploring one's own reaction to it. It is against this backdrop that grief has traditionally received much less attention in undergraduate training and beyond.

Where grief-education programmes for physicians do exist, focus has almost invariably been placed on the professional's role in reducing survivors' anxiety and how they communicate with those who are mourning. L. Sikstrom, 2019, in a review of 37 articles published between 1979 and 2019 and spanning multiple countries, found that most publications covered short voluntary training focused on ethical and legal issues in death and bereavement, and not physicians' own coping skills. The US Substance Abuse and Mental Health Services Administration (SAMHSA) in Maryland published a commendable pamphlet for physicians that started with instructions on 'identifying yourself and your role', before addressing behavioural aspects such as 'acknowledging the emotions of those who are suffering'. Ironically, the very first point presents the physician as an integral part of the grief process, and subsequent points serve to demonstrate why physician grief is often disenfranchised, as they are largely expected to 'rally on' without any focus on their own emotions. This lack of emotional outlet can, over time, affect mental health and job performance.

Many today are familiar with Kubler-Ross's traditional grief-process model, which moves through denial, anger, bargaining, depression and acceptance. While all grief shares some of **these** universal features, individual interruptions at critical stages can lead to complex grief syndromes that affect the body's biorhythms and physiological functioning. These disruptions increase the risk of obesity, burnout, depression, PTSD and addiction. Parallel initiatives, like those mentioned above for oncology nurses, are therefore also needed for clinicians. Tracking outcomes of these initiatives over time would offer invaluable data concerning how physicians process grief and consequently promote practices that improve their resilience.

A review by Li et al., 2023, found that while many articles support grief training throughout medical education there are few longitudinal studies over a significant time, so the actual impact of interventions on behaviour and practice in clinical settings is unclear. Also, among existing studies, group sizes have been small and methodologies largely do not reach the threshold for rigour, meaning limited valid conclusions can be drawn. Nevertheless, these articles together demonstrate that grief interventions can be wide and varied, depending on the individual's needs and cultural background. Approaches such as grief counseling, cognitive-behavioural therapy, art therapy and pharmacological interventions, to name but a few, can be particularly crucial for those who are at a higher risk of poor grief coping. This group clearly includes physicians.

Incorporating grief training into medical education faces a number of challenges. With faculty members lobbying for spots within the academic curriculum, grief-specific training in many universities is fragile, at best. Yet, it should not be assumed that clinicians somehow automatically know how to process feelings of loss. This realisation was made during the COVID-19 pandemic when, with high patient load and uncertainty about the new enemy, doctors' worries concerning their own health and that of their families often conflicted with their professional commitments. On top of this, patients died, often quite literally, while in their hands. It would be unnatural for clinicians not to be susceptible to the same grief reactions as their patients and patients' families.

Text 1: Questions 7–14

7. In Paragraph 1, the author mentions the different approaches to grief research in order to

    (A) applaud early researchers for their focus on this field of healthcare.

    (B) criticise the narrow focus of early researchers.

    (C) demonstrate the difficulty in focusing on so many different areas.

    (D) show how research in this area has evolved over time.

8. Morris and Block's suggestion that bereavement care is best tackled as a 'preventative model' refers to

    (A) educating the bereaved about different kinds of grief disorders.

    (B) preventing the physical symptoms that can occur during grief.

    (C) starting to tackle grief even before the dying person has passed away.

    (D) placing more focus on tackling grief when a death is expected.

9. Paragraph 3 suggests that doctors have traditionally had a certain approach to grief because

    (A) they associate grief with self-perceived failure to extend life.

    (B) they are so well-trained in diagnosis and effective treatment of disease.

    (C) medical schools do not consider grief a relevant topic.

    (D) most resources for training are allocated to other healthcare professions.

10. In the majority of the articles reviewed in Sikstrom's 2019 study

    (A) the most common topic was administrative processes surrounding death.

    (B) focus was placed on the same topics as in other programmes globally.

    (C) doctors were not obligated to attend grief-training programmes.

    (D) the data were insufficient to glean how effective grief training is.

11. The author thinks that the SAMHSA pamphlet

- (A) unintentionally highlights why physician grief can become complicated.
- (B) does not adequately address long-term physician-health issues.
- (C) falls short in educating physicians on how to counsel patients.
- (D) should have focused more on training workshops for physicians.

12. The word '**these**' in Paragraph 5 refers to

- (A) physical symptoms caused by grief.
- (B) the features of grief that are personal.
- (C) the normal evolution of grief.
- (D) the classic stages of grief.

13. In Paragraph 6, one limitation of the available data noted by the author is that

- (A) the studies were limited to descriptions of medical interventions.
- (B) the range of interventions studied were too wide.
- (C) studies did not identify those most at risk for complicated grief.
- (D) there is a lack of substantial prospective study data.

14. In Paragraph 7, the author is of the opinion that

- (A) doctors under pressure do not take their own need to mourn seriously.
- (B) it has taken too long for the emotional limitations of doctors to be acknowledged.
- (C) more research data is needed before doctors can access tools to help them cope with grief.
- (D) doctors do not fight hard enough for time and space to mourn and process their grief.

Text 2: Naturopathy

Naturopathy recognises the importance of balancing physical, mental and environmental factors for optimal health. Originating in Europe in the 16th to 17th centuries, and modernised in the 1900s, naturopahy principles include a belief in the body's ability to heal itself, removal of obstacles to healing, finding the underlying cause of illness and not just treating the symptoms, and they incorporate education and lifestyle changes with alternative and synthetic treatments. Naturopathic practitioners (NP) assess health and risk factors, and make appropriate interventions in partnership with their patients by using a range of therapies in a rational yet adaptable order. An NP may initially spend up to two hours understanding a patient's issues. As good communication between patient and healthcare professional is pivotal to improved health outcomes, the NP model, **at least in theory**, has prime opportunity to effect positive change in patient health.

Evidence-based medicine (EBM) differs from naturopathy in several key aspects. EBM consultations tend to be more hierarchal due, among other reasons, to doctors' time pressures. It focuses primarily on identifying disease and using established drugs, surgery and other interventions that do not take the individual into account and which have potential side effects that might be upsetting to those who are more anxious. While it is too simplistic to say that 'EBM treats the disease whereas naturopathy treats the patient', the medical doctor in EBM often controls decision-making when it comes to patient treatment, while the NP frames themself more as an educator and partner in healing. Although the naturopathy model may be less overwhelming or intimidating, it is still an unavoidable truth that EBM is equipped with proven treatments for a much wider range of illnesses. Acupuncture for post-surgical pain, aromatherapy for depression and diet for cardiovascular disease and type 2 diabetes are among the minority of naturopathic treatments that have some degree of supporting evidence. As these conditions are very common across populations, however, naturopathy remains a valid option still for many.

Despite licensing in many countries, the lack of consistent, reproducible scientific data on efficacy remains a key criticism for medical and researcher communities. Many naturopathic practices are not backed by randomised, double-blind controlled trials. Other therapies have been shown to be no more effective than a placebo, something that admittedly also occurs in scientific medicine. In the USA, phenylephrine, which has been an approved decongestant in nasal drops for years, is currently under consideration for recall as it has been shown to have no real effect. **This** cannot justify not requiring evidence in the naturopathy, however. All healthcare treatments should be informed by good science. It has, of course, been argued that randomised controlled trials do not fairly assess naturopathic therapies due to the holistic nature of naturopathy because patients cannot be blinded as to whether or not they meditate or do aromatherapy, and because outcomes are focused on general health rather than on an objective measurement such as blood pressure. 'Whole-systems research' is a possible alternative study approach as it evaluates within the context in which treatments are used and looks equally at qualitative and quantitative data.

Naturopathy also has risks. Diagnoses and therapies are often not standardised, which means that a patient may attribute their recovery to what is actually the natural cycle of a disorder or a placebo effect, and as treatments are based on the patient's unique experiences instead of conventional diagnostic criteria, hidden pathology could be missed. Prescribed diets may exclude whole food groups, causing potential nutritional deficiency, or prescribed supplements may lead to vitamin toxicity. Failure of patients to inform their medical doctor about alternative therapies they use may also pose a danger if the alternative therapies interfere with the normal functioning of pharmaceuticals.

All signs point to naturopathy and other alternative therapies not fading to the background any time soon. In 2012, Americans spent $14.7 billion on visits to complementary and integrative health practitioners such as chiropractors, acupuncturists, massage therapists and naturopaths, on top of a further $12.8 billion 'out-of-pocket' spend on natural products. This translates into 9.2% of all personal spending. A survey by the National Institute of Health revealed a jump in individuals using at least one of seven alternative medicine approaches, including yoga, meditation and pain management, from 19.2% in 2002 to 36.7% in 2022. It ought to be noted that the study coordinators admitted to there being issues in the study's design and its data collection, again highlighting the need for more rigorous proof of the effectiveness of alternative therapies. Patients should have the option to access a wide range of healthcare specialties, but they should also have access to enough high-quality information to make informed decisions, especially when considering treatment of legally and ethically high-stake conditions such as cardiovascular problems and cancer treatments.

The public's increasing uptake of alternative healthcare along with EBM means naturopathy could become a disruptive force in healthcare. To really become disruptive, alternative therapies must cure disease and transform the way in which medicine is practised over time. Naturopathy favours non-pharmacological health promotion, is cheaper than EBM, and naturopathic practitioners spend more time developing relationships with patients. These three factors could combine to change the economic dynamics of healthcare and win over patients, especially if health insurers cover more therapies in more countries.

Despite the lack of scientific validation for many naturopathy methods, evidence is not limited to randomised controlled trials. People also consider historical use, financial access and subjective feelings of well-being. As empirical observations are a valid source of information, individual case studies do constitute valid data. However, to solidify their credibility, naturopathic practitioners must contend with certain issues, including tackling unqualified practitioners who **co-opt** naturopathic medicine and devalue its legitimate philosophy, and publishing findings from harder data on efficacy.

15. In Paragraph 1, the use of the phrase **'at least in theory'** suggests that the author

- (A) has doubts concerning how long NPs actually spend with patients.
- (B) is ambivalent about whether or not NPs achieve better health outcomes.
- (C) approves of the use of alternative therapies over modern medical treatments.
- (D) doubts the superior quality of communication between NPs and patients.

16. In Paragraph 2, the author makes the general point that

- (A) the disease focus of EBM is too narrow and not individualised enough.
- (B) a large number of patients could benefit from naturopathy.
- (C) having the medical doctor decide what treatments to give is restrictive.
- (D) EBM is not necessarily as effective as one would expect.

17. **'This'** in Paragraph 3 refers to

- (A) an example of ineffective ingredients in accepted medicines.
- (B) the inclusion of unscientific therapies in NP practice.
- (C) acceptance of naturopathy therapies by health insurers.
- (D) the scientific research that underpins cough medication.

18. The main purpose of Paragraph 4 is to

- (A) educate readers on how to ensure an accurate diagnosis.
- (B) persuade readers to avoid naturopathic therapies and diets.
- (C) educate readers about specific herb-drug interactions.
- (D) help readers make informed decisions about alternative therapies.

19. In Paragraph 5, deficiencies in the study's methods are mentioned in order to

   (A) show that the National Institute of Health is generally not a reliable data source.

   (B) show that the survey focused on the wrong issues.

   (C) reiterate the ongoing problems with getting data on alternative therapies.

   (D) reinforce the importance of accurate data on heart and cancer treatments.

20. Paragraph 6 suggests that naturopathy could become disruptive as it could potentially

   (A) displace the current stakeholders and value system.

   (B) upset patients' confidence in its effectiveness.

   (C) force medical and alternative practitioners to work as a team.

   (D) interfere with securing whole-person healthy outcomes.

21. Based on the final paragraph, the writer thinks that

   (A) empirical data about naturopathy is just as valuable as randomised control trials.

   (B) the general public has broader definitions for what it accepts as proof.

   (C) more needs to be done to assess and recall established-but-ineffective drugs.

   (D) cost considerations are the main force driving people to use complementary medicine.

22. In the final paragraph, '**co-opt**' means

   (A) demand to be recognised as partners.

   (B) join legitimate naturopathy associations.

   (C) misuse the naturopathy title.

   (D) take over the field.

End of Part C

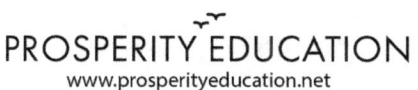

Occupational English Test

Reading

Test 2

Part A

- Look at the four texts (**A–D**) in the accompanying **text booklet**.
- For each question (**1–20**) look through the texts (**A–D**) to find the relevant information.
- Write your answers in the spaces provided in this **question paper**.
- Answer all the questions within the 15-minute time limit.
- Your answers should **only** be taken from texts **A–D** and must be correctly spelt.

Neonatal Conjunctivitis: Questions

Questions 1–7

For each question (**1–7**), decide which text (**A, B, C** or **D**) the information comes from. Write the letter **A, B, C** or **D** in the space provided. You may use any letter more than once.

In which text can you find information about

1 why babies are vulnerable to conjunctivitis complications? _____

2 choices for topical eye treatment? _____

3 incubation period of different kinds of neonatal conjunctivitis? _____

4 how babies become infected? _____

5 details of at-home eye care routine for neonatal conjunctivitis? _____

6 baby weight issues that can occur with maternal microbial infections? _____

7 rates for maternal-to-baby transmission for different infections? _____

Questions 8–14

Answer each of the questions (**8–14**) with a word or short phrase from one of the texts. Each answer may include words, numbers or both. You should **not** write full sentences.

8 What is the minimum daily dose of ceftriaxone that can be given?

_____

9 When should a specialist referral occur on diagnosing neonatal conjunctivitis?

_____

10 Where in a baby's body can C. trachomatis live without causing illness?

_____

11 In confirmed maternal STI infection, what should be discussed besides caesarean section?

_____

12 What proportion of living neonates develop neonatal conjunctivitis?

_____

13 What can happen to the cornea in C. trachomatis infection?

_____

14 What must you not do when treating neonatal conjunctivitis?

_____

Questions 15–20

Complete each of the sentences (**15–20**) with a word or short phrase from one of the texts. Each answer may include words, numbers or both.

15 _____ is a microbe that rapidly infects inside the eye and can cause fatality.

16 Babies can receive ceftriaxone if they were born at or after _____.

17 When cleansing a baby's eyes, cleansing motion should be _____.

18 Babies can pick up the infection from the mother's _____.

19 Babies receiving recommended treatment for C. trachomatis could show signs of _____.

20 In HSV infection, the thin discharge coming from the eyes is sometimes _____.

End of Part A

Neonatal Conjunctivitis: Texts

Text A

Overview

Neonatal conjunctivitis (also called ophthalmia neonatorum) occurs in 1–2% of total live births and symptoms present during the first month of life. The condition has non-infectious and microbial causes. Aseptic conjunctivitis is caused by chemicals, especially silver nitrate solution which has been long used as prophylaxis for gonococcal ophthalmia but which has now been mostly replaced by modern topical antibiotics. Silver nitrate solutions are still used in some high-incidence settings.

Aetiology

Infectious conjunctivitis is either bacterial or viral in origin. The maternal cervix and urethra act as reservoirs for microbes, and conjunctivitis is acquired during the birthing transition. Chlamydia trachomatis is the most common bacterial cause and appears from day 5–14 after birth.

Neisseria gonorrhoea infection is the second most common but causes the most severe complications. It usually appears 2–5 days after birth but can take up to 14 days.

Staphylococcus, streptococcus, Enterobacter, *E. coli*, and, rarely, pseudomonas account for most of the remaining incidences. Viral neonatal conjunctivitis accounts for just 1% of cases and is associated with the herpes simplex virus, taking 6–14 days before clinical disease is evident. More rarely, adenoviruses may cause neonatal conjunctivitis.

Text B

Clinical Features and Prognosis

The conjunctiva becomes inflamed with dilated blood vessels and excessive eye secretions. As newborns have immature immune systems and do not produce tears until they are over two weeks old, infections can cause long-term complications if not promptly and properly treated.

Neisseria gonorrhoea

- Have severe bilateral purulent conjunctival discharge
- Spread to the nose, meninges and blood
- Severe complications include corneal ulceration, anterior chamber perforation, and blindness

Chlamydia trachomatis

- Infection may appear mild with little redness and a serous discharge, or may be severe with swelling of the conjunctiva (chemosis)
- Neovascularisation can form over the cornea, causing blindness (rare occurrence)
- Can spread to ears causing otitis, and also to lungs, causing life-threatening pneumonia
- Asymptomatic colonisation of the throat and rectum is common

Herpes Simplex Virus

- Produces periorbital vesicles with swollen eyelids and moderately red conjunctiva; eye discharge is thin and may be slightly bloody
- Eye problems can worsen due to corneal ulceration (keratitis)
- Further spread can result in encephalitis or meningitis

Other bacterial infections

- Antenatal complications include low gestational weight and pre-term birth
- Postnatal complications include low birth weight
- Pseudomonas quickly develops into intra-orbital infection – can cause death; requires fast and aggressive treatment

Chemicals

- Eyelid swelling, redness and discharge (watery, mucous or purulent)
- Settles with regular irrigation using sterile normal saline

Text C

Management

Obtain cervical and neonatal eyes swabs, plus full blood panel. Start empirical treatment pending culture results: clean eyes frequently with copious 0.9% isotonic saline. For gonococcal and chlamydial infection, the application of topical 0.5% erythromycin and 1% tetracycline ointments are considered equally effective (available in single-dose preparations). For other bacterial infections, topical silver nitrate, povidone-iodine or erythromycin are all effective for prophylaxis. Do not patch eyes. Same-day paediatric or ophthalmology consultation required. Daily monitoring.

Causative agent	Treatment of clinical infection, cause confirmed
Chemical	Non-specific. Eye toilet done regularly. Observe for suspected super-imposed microbial infection (purulent discharge, febrile and ill-looking baby)
N. gonorrhoea	Single dose *ceftriaxone 25–50mg/kg/24hr to a maximum of 125mg Alternative: single-dose cefotaxime 100mg/kg
C. trachomatis	Oral **erythromycin 50mg/kg/24hr divided in 4 doses for 14 days. A second course often required to fully treat nasopharyngeal infection
HSV	IV acyclovir 60mg/kg/day divided in 3 doses, given 14–21 days HSV keratitis treated with 0.15% ganciclovir or 1% trifluridine drops (max. 9 drops in 24 hours).
Pseudomonas & other microbes	If pseudomonas suspected, start empirical treatment immediately Oral **erythromycin 50mg/kg/24hr divided in 4 doses for 14 days OR oral azithromycin 20mg/kg once daily for 3 days Regimen may change based on culture sensitivity results

*Ceftriaxone contraindicated in babies with gestation <41 weeks, especially if jaundiced or on calcium-containing solutions.

**Erythromycin associated with development of pyloric stenosis. Observe baby closely.

Text D

Guidance to be Provided to Parents

Prenatal

- Regular maternal prenatal appointments advised
- Discuss sexual and reproductive history, and possibility of sexually transmitted infections
- Educate about vertical transmission of pathogens during vaginal delivery (foetal risk of infection in active maternal genital herpes is up to 60%. In maternal chlamydia or gonorrhoea, is over 25%.)
- Include screening for N. gonorrhoea and C. trachomatis in routine prenatal work ups, in addition to other relevant STIs, e.g. syphilis. Test sexual partner(s), if possible.
- If high maternal risk of infection, discuss cesarean section. (C-section recommended in active genital herpes infection.)
- If maternal infection confirmed: also discuss drug treatment options

Postnatal (ideally discussed before maternal discharge)

Discuss timeline to clinical signs of neonatal conjunctivitis and possible need for hospitalisation depending on cause and severity. Reassure parent(s) of good response to treatment.

If clinical infection occurs and in-patient management is necessary, have parent(s) observe staff and learn eye-toilet routine: handwashing, wearing gloves, eye irrigation, eye wiping in direction from nose to ear, use one cotton ball for one wipe only and correct handling or disposal of care items.

Stress: Always wash hands before and after eye care. Handle baby's items separately from other domestic items. Minimise contact with others in the household until confirmation of resolved infection. Attend recommended follow-up appointments.

End of Part A | Text booklet

Part B

In this part of the test, there are six short extracts relating to the work of health professionals. For questions **1–6**, choose the answer (**A**, **B** or **C**) that you think fits best according to the text.

Your answers should be made by filling in the circle completely:

1. The memo states that teeth containing amalgam

    (A) should not be returned to patients.

    (B) may be used for teaching students.

    (C) can be handled like teeth without amalgam.

| To: Dental Staff |
Re: Handling Of Extracted Teeth
Extracted teeth may be contaminated with potentially infectious material and must be handled in keeping with Occupational Safety Regulations (OSR).
Teeth without amalgam must be discarded in regulated medical waste containers for incineration. Teeth containing amalgam should not be placed with regulated medical waste. Instead, they can be disposed of through local metal-recycling agencies according to their agency's policies.
Extracted teeth to be used for preclinical training must be cleaned of all blood and debris and stored or transported in leakproof, clearly-labeled biohazard containers until sterilisation.
Sterilisation methods include applying heat or, for amalgam containing teeth, soaking in 10% formalin for two weeks.
Teeth not containing amalgam are preferred for educational use.
Extracted teeth can be returned to patients upon request. Once taken by the patient, the teeth are no longer subject to OSR.

2. When adjusting a patient's restraint order

   (A) the physician must first see the patient face-to-face.

   (B) the padding holding the limbs should be changed.

   (C) patients should be continuously watched for 30 minutes.

To: Nursing Staff

MEMO: Use Of Mechanical Restraints

When there is imminent danger of harm to a patient themselves or to others, nursing staff must inform the medical officer in charge who then assesses and documents the need for physical restraints, including the nature and duration of the restraints.

The medical officer must assess the patient within the first hour of restraint placement and, at the end of this period, update the order following an in-person evaluation.

Restraints should ideally be applied to the patient lying on a bed, with both arms and legs tied with soft bandages. They should be constantly monitored by trained personnel throughout the restraint time or, if this is not possible, be visualised for the first 15 minutes then every 15 minutes thereafter for physical condition, mental comfort and fitness for removal of restraints.

Physical restraints should not be used longer than absolutely necessary, and never as a punishment or to counter staff shortages.

3. According to the guidelines, a professional interpreter

   (A) is only needed when a patient refuses the services of a friend or family member.

   (B) should be present to advise on the extent of the language barrier.

   (C) must be used at some point when communicating with the patient.

Elective Admissions: Best Practice For Patients Needing Interpreters

Patients with limited English (LEP) should always be offered the service of an interpreter at the start of an interview. Using friends and family as interpreters should be avoided except in cases of minor emergencies, as this can lead to poor interpretation of medical terms, deliberate censoring of information or patient distress at loved ones learning sensitive details.

Educate the patient about the advantages of a professional interpreter, that strict confidentiality is maintained and that they may request a male or female interpreter. This initial information must be conveyed using a professional interpreter to ensure that the patient clearly understands their communication options. If the patient refuses the service, reevaluate the safety of continuing care given the extent of the language barrier. Details of the information given to the patient, the patient's final decision and the justification for any care actions should all be documented.

4. The smoking policy emphasises that

   (A) staff must remove their uniforms before smoking regular or e-cigarettes.

   (B) staff are not allowed to leave hospital premises during their shift to smoke.

   (C) patients who insist on smoking will be instead treated at home.

To: Nursing Staff
Subject: Smoking

Smoking tobacco products, including e-cigarettes, is not allowed anywhere on hospital premises.

Staff are not entitled to extra time for smoking breaks. Instances of staff repeatedly taking too-frequent breaks or breaks not agreed to with the team manager may be escalated to the Director of Nursing. Staff should never smoke in uniform, while wearing their ID badge or when representing the hospital in an official capacity. It is not acceptable for staff to simply cover their uniform with a coat when smoking.

Patients who smoke should receive brief counselling from a doctor, nurse or trained professional. Patients who still insist on smoking on hospital premises, and become aggressive when approached, should be advised that such conduct could result in them being asked to leave hospital premises.

5. The purpose of the memo is to

   (A) educate link workers on the function of social prescribers.

   (B) highlight statistical data about real social needs of older persons.

   (C) help clinical facilities to update their patient-management approach.

Memo: Social Prescribing

The practice of social prescribing recognises that determinants of health include poverty, isolation and loneliness. Non-medical staff, called 'link workers', work within the social-prescribing framework to support individuals in accessing community resources and services that address social, emotional and practical needs. They act as intermediaries between patients and the community, helping to bridge gaps that traditional medical care may not address.

The initiative was prompted by the results of the recent regional census which revealed that 23% of respondents over 67 years old cite loneliness and transportation difficulties as major issues affecting their social and mental health.

The attached toolkit is geared toward GP practices, long-term care and other care facilities, and provides details of the role and range of available regional services, a list of social prescribers and guidelines on how to incorporate social prescribing into your healthcare model. Any member of a healthcare team can suggest referral to a social prescriber.

6. The training information cautions that

    (A) formal training is not required after the Triage Programme.

    (B) hospital emergency resources were wasted in the past.

    (C) the Emergency Department used to experience the most lawsuits.

Becoming An Emergency Department Triage Nurse
Nurses with a 3- or 4-year nursing degree and a minimum of 24 months' full-time work as a registered nurse may be considered for the Emergency Department Triage Nurse Programme, which includes: • a 12-hour theory course including the Emergency Severity Index for patient categorisation • simulation room and role-play practice • shadowing of and supervision by an experienced triage nurse. After triage certification, triage nurses must regularly submit proof of renewed skills in related subjects such as Advanced Cardiac Life Support, among others, in order to maintain their accreditation. Triage is critical to ensure patients access the right care at the right time, and that hospital resources are used optimally. Historically, ER triage resulted in the highest rates for litigation across all clinical departments. Rigorous certification protocols have reversed this trend.

End of Part B

Part C

In this part of the test, there are two texts about different aspects of healthcare. For questions **7–22**, choose the answer (**A**, **B**, **C** or **D**) that you think fits best according to the text.

Your answers should be made by filling in the circle completely: Ⓐ Ⓑ ⓒ Ⓓ

Text 1: Dengue

About half of the world's population is now at risk of dengue fever, with roughly 200–400 million infections diagnosed annually, yet there continues to be no specific treatment. The dengue virus is spread by the Aedes mosquito species, and the infection itself has a wide spectrum of symptomatology and severity. The vast majority of those infected will have no symptoms or mild symptoms that are often mistaken by patients and their primary care providers for illnesses such as the common cold or influenza. These patients commonly use over-the-counter or other home-treatments, experience no significant loss in daily productivity and their real diagnoses remain undocumented. At the other end of the spectrum is the minority of infected persons who develop severe dengue and require hospitalisation.

To further complicate dengue's clinical picture, individuals who become infected for the second time are at greater risk of severe dengue, which can be fatal. The World Health Organization (WHO) has estimated that out of 390 million dengue virus infections, 96 million cases manifest clinically. The high number of infections, and the fact that milder versions are generally the norm, has helped to create **a double-edged sword** with respect to developing strategies for monitoring, vector control and the treatment of severe forms of the infection. Historically, dengue typically received limited investment as the disease burden was previously restricted to underserved settings. However, the complexity of the disease has recently prompted much interest from various research teams that all want to win the race to find a solution.

There were 500,000 confirmed dengue infections in 2000. In 2023, there were 6.5 million infections resulting in over 7000 related deaths and, perhaps more alarmingly, the profile of dengue spread had changed. The Aedes mosquito vector is no longer confined to tropical and subtropical countries but increasingly is found in Europe, the USA and the Mediterranean. Raised global temperatures, rainfall and humidity provide conditions that encourage the mosquito to spread to new regions. Additionally, political instability and mass migration give rise to poor housing with overcrowded conditions, while financial disenfranchisement can lead to mass homelessness even in societies that are not in conflict. Even in more stable homes, poor awareness and practice with respect to water storage, plant-keeping and self-protection against mosquito bites can all impact the risk of the disease.

Factors contributing to dengue rates are not identical across all countries. A 2018 hospital-based study in India, for instance, revealed that there is no longer even distribution throughout the year. Dengue reporting has shifted mostly to the Indian monsoon months of June to December, and those who spent more time at home during the day showed higher rates of infection than those who left home daily for work. While there was some awareness among people of dengue-prevention methods, with common behaviours including spraying the skin at bedtime and using bed nets, the dengue mosquito is increasingly more active during the day and so this gap in knowledge needs to be corrected. Furthermore, the study found that distance from healthcare and cultural beliefs contributed to delays in seeking medical help in situations where timely diagnosis and case reporting are vital to control spread.

In Peru, the 2023 outbreak severely impacted the capital city, Lima, whereas historically, numbers were driven by infections in the Amazon rainforest regions. One possible contributing factor to this could be the deficient water system in Peru. Unreliable flowing water in the outskirts of urban areas, longer hot seasons and heavy rains together could have resulted in more stagnant water, precipitating a surge in mosquito numbers and consequent dengue outbreak. Meanwhile, in Florida in the USA, a 2022 study suggested that while previous outbreaks were assumed to be from imported cases, there seemed instead to be endemic circulation in certain hotspots within the state.

With no specific treatment, focus is on vector control and vaccines. Releasing populations of modified mosquitoes with a reduced capacity for carrying the dengue virus has sometimes been shown to be both biologically and cost-effective, and it has the added advantage of not completely eradicating the mosquito and thus maintaining environmental balance. However, one anomaly noted in Singapore, which saw a successful introduction of local vector, was a paradoxical increase in the number of dengue outbreaks in the country. This was hypothesised to be due to lowered herd immunity to virus variants. This example surely underlines the need for ensuring that vector control must be integrated into a wider coordinated approach.

Another issue is that currently approved vaccines are for those who have had one dengue infection and are at risk of severe dengue if reinfected. Despite the clear clinical value, the vaccine does not therefore have the expected attribute of whole-population use. Even though the perfect dengue vaccine that protects everyone from all dengue variants is not yet imminent, the currently approved vaccines do effectively immunise some people who are a part of the disease burden, even if only a niche group.

It is not only Aedes vector numbers and vaccine coverage that should be closely monitored. Currently, the primary mode of virus transmission between humans requires the mosquito, but vertical transmission during pregnancy is known to occur, linked to the timing of infection during pregnancy. This vertical transmission, which can result in pre-term birth, low birthweight and foetal distress, exists, but is as rare as transmission via blood products, organ donation and transfusions. However, the mosquito is highly adaptable and, with the capacity of viruses to mutate, vigilance and ongoing vigorous public education must include awareness of potentially dangerous changes in direction of both virus and vector activity.

Text 1: Questions 7–14

7. The purpose of the Paragraph 1 is to

    (A) show why the disease might be unreported.

    (B) show how varied symptoms are.

    (C) to raise awareness of how many people are affected.

    (D) to raise awareness of how dangerous the disease is.

8. The term '**double-edged sword**' refers to

    (A) two similar categories of problems.

    (B) both positive and negative aspects of tackling the infection.

    (C) the infection possibly occurring twice in the same individual.

    (D) the sheer danger the infection represents to populations.

9. In Paragraph 3, that author suggests that

    (A) multiple tiers in society are responsible for dengue spread.

    (B) war contributes disproportionately to dengue spread.

    (C) those fleeing political unrest bring the dengue vector with them.

    (D) human activities have pushed the mosquito out of its natural habitat.

10. The author gives the information on India in Paragraph 4 to

    (A) encourage people not to stay home during the daytime.

    (B) instruct on exactly when to implement dengue measures.

    (C) show why some cultural beliefs need to be stopped.

    (D) demonstrate specific situations where education is needed.

11. In Paragraph 5, '**this**' refers to

- (A) Peru having a history of endemic dengue in cities.
- (B) the occurrence of dengue in the Amazon regions.
- (C) the poor supply of fresh water within the city.
- (D) the distribution of the 2023 outbreak in Peru.

12. The writer describes the situation in Singapore as 'paradoxical' because

- (A) the country was unable to manufacture vaccines locally.
- (B) the country used methods that did not effectively control the vector population.
- (C) decreasing the numbers of mosquitoes in some ways did more harm than good.
- (D) Singapore focused too strongly on vector control instead of a multi-disciplined approach.

13. In Paragraph 7, the writer contends that

- (A) it is taking too long for a more widely applicable vaccine to be approved.
- (B) protecting even a small percentage of persons from dengue is a significant achievement.
- (C) that those who have been infected already should not be prioritised for vaccines.
- (D) that the cost of developing a vaccine against all dengue variants would be too burdensome.

14. In the final paragraph, the writer

- (A) worries that the virus may find new ways to spread.
- (B) is surprised by the range of ways the virus can spread.
- (C) is pleased that maternal-child transmission is not a major contributor.
- (D) thinks not enough attention is being paid to special demographics.

Text 2: Multicultural Healthcare Teams

The modern trend of accelerated globalisation has seen an increased diversity in the national and cultural backgrounds of not only patients but their healthcare teams as well. However, conflicts can arise when people from such diverse backgrounds are brought together in pressurised situations. In the context of the workplace, these conflicts can result in dysfunctional team dynamics and sub-optimal collaboration. Yet, despite the high levels of interdependence in health teams and the clear implications for patient care, there are still not many studies specifically on the impacts of multiculturalism within healthcare teams and how to effectively tackle issues that might arise. **This** can be attributed to it being a relatively new global issue, the focus on traditional determinants of health and the complexity of tracking, collecting data and reproducing similar studies on multicultural conflicts within health teams.

Conflicts can result from preconceptions about training and knowledge level, fear of liability if a mistake is made and legitimate workload pressures that make staff orientation difficult which, in turn, can increase the occurrence of mistakes. Misinterpretation of language used and of the emotion or intent behind it can also occur. Additionally, patients may express a clear preference for someone who looks or speaks like them, presenting supervisors with the challenge of personnel re-allocation in the face of the established links between patient satisfaction, compliance and recovery. If not acknowledged and addressed, negative team experiences can result in deficiencies in professional skills, increased burden on the remaining members of the team leading to delays, omissions or duplications in patient care, and even breaches in professional codes of conduct. Conversely, a 2015 study by Lyubovnikova et al. noted that hospitals in which staff report higher levels of teamwork and management of interdependencies have lower rates of workplace injuries and illnesses, fewer reports of harassment and violence are made, and fewer staff express a plan to leave the organisation.

Overall, diversity in clinical teams has been shown to be positively associated with improved healthcare quality. At the patient level, care in which clinician and patient share an attribute such as ethnicity, religion, language or gender is associated with improved communication, medication adherence and, ultimately, enhanced patient satisfaction and health outcomes. Against this backdrop of study data are the professionals giving personal accounts of conflicts within healthcare teams stemming from religion, ethnicity, gender- or native-language-disparities. These subjective perspectives are not scientific proof, but the sheer volume of recounts warrants quantitative study into the exact scope of the problem and possible solutions given the high stakes for those involved. In a US nationwide survey during March and April 2022, the results of 15 in-depth interviews with registered nurses demonstrated the mental-health toll caused by poor teamwork and that this was forcing some nurses from the profession. Even in 2015, Tuttas already noted that perceived discrimination was one of the key barriers to successful staff recruitment and retention of diverse nurses.

Research on the effects of increasing workplace diversity and multiculturalism has grown, but the healthcare industry lags behind. Other business sectors show that there is more innovation, better team communication, improved adaptability to change and better risk-assessment skills in teams that are more diverse. A link has even been demonstrated between diversity and improved financial performance. Meanwhile, the few existing healthcare studies at least show that patients fare better overall when care is provided by more diverse teams. There is definite value in seeing how similar indices play out in healthcare settings that must also remain financially viable. However, there are many unique research questions and kinds of data to be collected, and even more will emerge as healthcare catches up with other sectors.

Institutional leadership sets the tone within institutions, and has a prime position to collect data, advance areas for more study and implement change. However, top-down hierarchy can also inhibit frank two-way communication and can represent a **conflict of interest** in the growth of an institution. So far, healthcare-institution leaders have had to make decisions about team-building based on studies from other sectors that include conflicting findings about the association between factors. Nevertheless, much can be learned from studying healthcare teams as singular entities. They are fertile ground for the observation of unique interpersonal dynamics and different team types, and they offer opportunities for large-scale testing of theories. Moreover, the talent pool of professionals with heterogeneous backgrounds and problem-solving skills are well-placed to solve healthcare issues prevalent within their own cultural demographic.

Another thing to focus on is the need for training healthcare institutions in capacity-building, which is defined as the development and strengthening of resources that institutions need to adapt to and thrive in amidst periods of change. This includes increasing competences and developing training for specific issues that are not currently being addressed. Interestingly, a crucial 2019 European Union study by Chiarenza et al. found that most existing training programs are poorly linked to key organisational functions, and that the ones that do feature these largely focus on responses in emergencies as opposed to being proactive in problem-solving. The study was focused on the care of patients from diverse cultural backgrounds, but arguably training concepts are transferable to training the multicultural health teams on how they function themselves. Capacity-building should encompass the entire team, from leaders and educators to students at undergraduate and post-graduate levels, and could even include mandatory continuous education accreditations in multiculturalism.

There is no turning back the clock on global migration. Researchers must build earnest momentum in gathering, collating and sharing data on the dynamics and impact of multicultural healthcare teams. At the leadership level, research on patient care impact and return on investment requires evidence to correctly guide strategy and goal achievement. Training in working side-by-side with colleagues from diverse backgrounds is needed to help improve employee morale and decrease staff turnover. Furthermore, considering the importance of team-functioning in patient care, human resource departments (HRD) may need to move away from hiring solely on the basis of academic qualifications and staffing numbers, and incorporate applicant experience with multicultural training, especially if the financial-performance findings from other sectors hold true for healthcare settings.

15. 'This' in Paragraph 1 refers to

- (A) the impact on patient care.
- (B) conflicts within multicultural teams.
- (C) the interdependence of team members.
- (D) the lack of studies on team multiculturalism.

16. In Paragraph 2, the author suggests that

- (A) preconceptions about professionals from a different background are without merit.
- (B) there is some merit to giving patients the kind of staff member they want.
- (C) there is seldom a valid reason for not orientating new staff correctly.
- (D) staff members should be trained in what is appropriate to say.

17. The author mentions the Lyubovinikova study to

- (A) demonstrate the wide personal and professional impacts of good teamwork.
- (B) indicate how to better manage staff taking sick leave.
- (C) show how hospitals can leave themselves vulnerable to employee lawsuits.
- (D) show how staff help each other when there are good team dynamics.

18. In Paragraph 3, the outcome of the interview with 15 nurses was given to highlight

- (A) how few nurses were willing to speak about details of their ordeals.
- (B) how few nurses in the survey experienced truly negative environments.
- (C) how individual experience can impact the wider sector.
- (D) the exact nature of the difficulties the nurses experienced.

19. In Paragraph 4, the author is of the opinion that other business sectors

- (A) show how much should be invested in healthcare team research.
- (B) provide a good template for a healthcare model.
- (C) demonstrate more innovation in designing research studies.
- (D) have little to offer healthcare research as the settings are too different.

20. The author uses the term '**conflict of interest**' to reflect that

- (A) the power structure might inhibit the goals they want to achieve.
- (B) issues in other sectors are transferable to healthcare.
- (C) researchers are conflicted about doing healthcare-team studies.
- (D) researchers are interested in only one kind of healthcare-team study.

21. In Paragraph 6, capacity-building is described as important for healthcare institutions because it

- (A) will identify specific reasons for team conflict.
- (B) helps organisations spell out their key functions.
- (C) helps organisations deal with emergencies more quickly.
- (D) allows for development of intercultural skills.

22. In the final paragraph, the author asserts that

- (A) hiring decisions should be guided by commercial revenue data.
- (B) leaders, staff and HRD need research data before creating training programmes.
- (C) priority should be given to research on financial performance.
- (D) institutions should not make changes until evidence-based research is available.

End of Part C

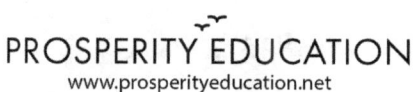

Occupational English Test

Reading

Test 3

Part A

- Look at the four texts (**A–D**) in the accompanying **text booklet**.
- For each question (**1–20**) look through the texts (**A–D**) to find the relevant information.
- Write your answers in the spaces provided in this **question paper**.
- Answer all the questions within the 15-minute time limit.
- Your answers should **only** be taken from texts **A–D** and must be correctly spelt.

Tuberculosis in Children up to 5 Years Old: Questions

Questions 1–7

For each question (**1–7**), decide which text (**A, B, C** or **D**) the information comes from. Write the letter **A, B, C** or **D** in the space provided. You may use any letter more than once.

In which text can you find information about

1. how to treat TB when there is concomitant HIV? _____

2. how administration of medication will be overseen? _____

3. the stages of TB infection in children? _____

4. specific findings in the different diagnostic tests? _____

5. what to do if a test is negative? _____

6. drug contraindications? _____

7. kinds of specimens to be tested in suspected TB? _____

Questions 8–14

Answer each of the questions (**8–14**) with a word or short phrase from one of the texts. Each answer may include words, numbers or both. You should **not** write full sentences.

8. What specific method is favoured for TB skin testing in children younger than 5 years old?

   _____

9. Where in the long bones is affected by TB?

   _____

10 When there is no direct healthcare supervision, what can a father do to ensure correct timing of medication?

_____

11 Which drug is contraindicated in inactive TB?

_____

12 In active TB, what proportion of bacteria culture samples show positive results?

_____

13 What is the maximum amount of pyrazinamide that can be given?

_____

14 How much more likely is TB infection to be found in persons with HIV?

_____

Questions 15–20

Complete each of the sentences (15–20) with a word or short phrase from one of the texts. Each answer may include words, numbers or both.

15 The cough of children with TB is described as _____.

16 On a negative TB blood test, guardians should receive further disease information and _____.

17 Caregivers should watch for previously healthy contacts who develop poor eating habits that cause _____.

18 To help patients take the treatment as directed, the _____ should be chosen.

19 Combinations of drugs can now be obtained as _____.

20 Besides disease exacerbation, _____ can also develop if medication is missed.

End of Part A

Tuberculosis in Children Up to 5 Years Old: Texts

Text A

Overview

Mycobacterium tuberculosis is spread via droplets released during coughing, laughing, sneezing, speaking or singing. Tuberculosis (TB) is not likely to be spread through casual contact with personal items or shared use of a toilet.

Features

Infected children have atypical or varied presentations that make diagnosis challenging. Children are more likely than adults to develop active, extrapulmonary or miliary TB spread through the blood stream. However, most children have few symptoms besides a brassy cough. Extrapulmonary TB can present with lymphadenitis (scrofula), involvement of the vertebrae (Pott's disease) or growth points of long bones, meningitis, or involvement of kidneys or other organs. Risk of infection is especially high if children have immune deficits or live in close situations where TB is prevalent. Those with the human immunodeficiency virus have an eighteen-times-higher risk of contracting TB.

The three stages of TB include exposure, latency and active disease.

Immediately following exposure to bacteria from someone with TB, the child has no symptoms and tests are negative. Once the bacteria are in the body, they are deactivated by a healthy immune system and the child will have no symptoms. For many children, TB remains at this latent stage for life but can become active TB and, without treatment, become severe and the child can spread the infection to others. TB can be fatal.

Investigation Profile

In latent TB, skin tests will be positive, but chest X-rays will be normal and the child will not be able to spread infection to others. Diagnostic tests are positive in active TB.

Text B

Assessment Protocol

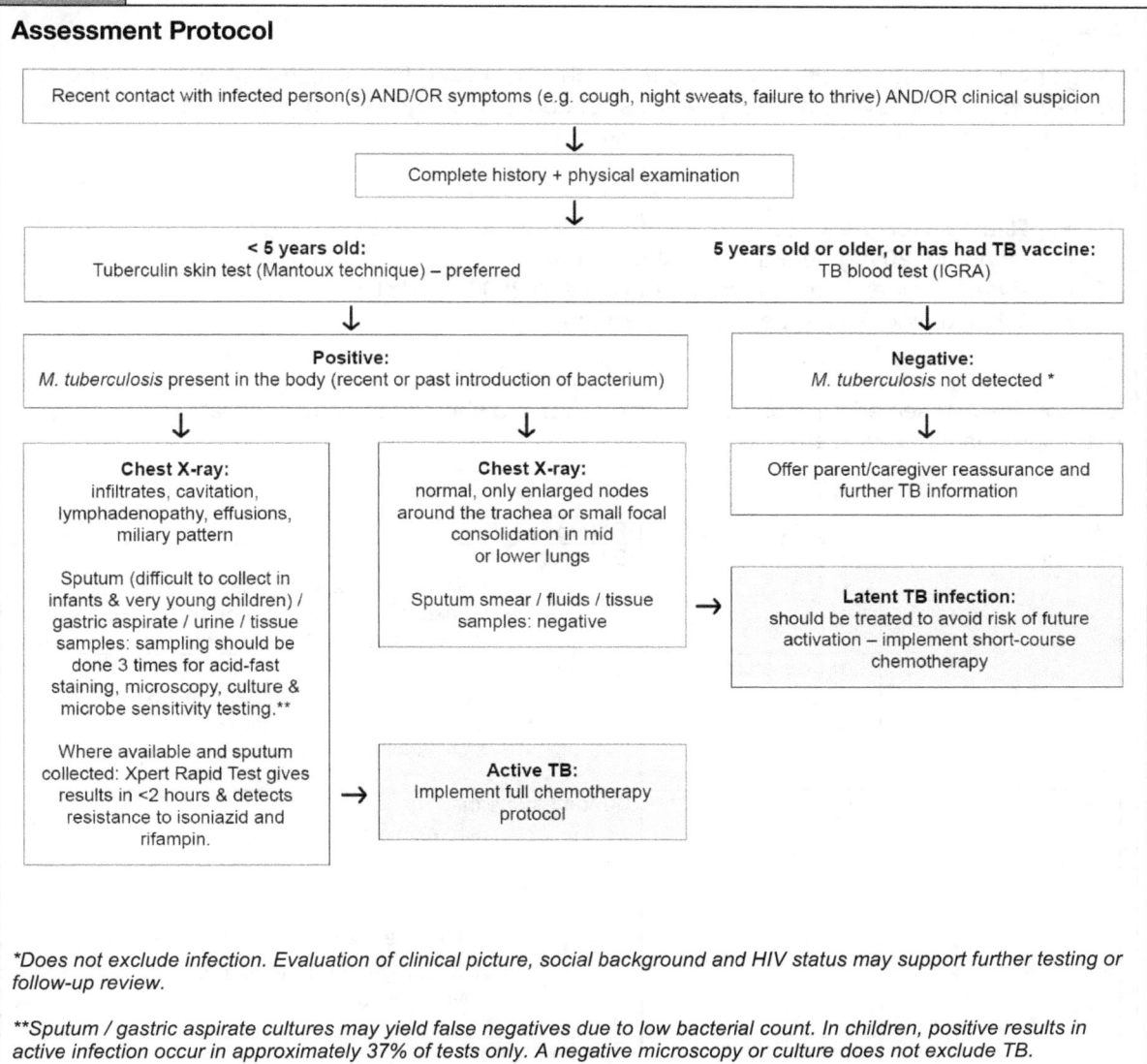

*Does not exclude infection. Evaluation of clinical picture, social background and HIV status may support further testing or follow-up review.

**Sputum / gastric aspirate cultures may yield false negatives due to low bacterial count. In children, positive results in active infection occur in approximately 37% of tests only. A negative microscopy or culture does not exclude TB.

Text C

Medication Protocols

Drugs must be dosed strictly according to weight. Pre-mixed formulations are now available for multi-drug regimens. Where appropriate, assist compliance by choosing the shortest protocol. The 4 first-line drugs in short programmes are 'RIPE':

- **R**ifampin (or weekly form, rifapentine): 20 mg per kg, up to 600 mg daily
- **I**soniazid: 20 mg per kg, up to 400 mg daily
- **P**yrazinamide: 40 mg per kg (not to exceed 2000 mg daily)
- **E**thionamide: 20 mg per kg, up to 750 mg daily

Bedaquiline is reserved for multi-drug resistant TB and should not be used in latent, extrapulmonary or drug-sensitive TB.

Type	Drug Resistance	Regimen
Latent	none	Either of <ul><li>daily rifampin x 4 months</li><li>weekly rifapentine x 4 months</li><li>daily isoniazid x 6-12 months</li></ul>
	drug-resistant	Either of <ul><li>weekly isoniazid + rifapentine x 3 months</li><li>daily rifampin x 4 months</li><li>daily isoniazid plus rifampin x 3 months</li></ul>
Pulmonary	none	4 months of either <ul><li>Isoniazid & rifampin only</li></ul> or <ul><li>In HIV prevalence – all 4 first-line drugs (RIPE) together. Extend to 6 months in severe disease.</li></ul>
	drug-resistant	Special regimen: <ul><li>bedaquiline x 6 months plus ethionamide, isoniazid, pyrazinamide with added ethambutol, levofloxacin, and clofazimine x 4 months</li></ul> Then: <ul><li>ethambutol, pyrazinamide, levofloxacin and clofazimine x 5 months</li></ul>
Extrapulmonary TB	–	Either of <ul><li>isoniazid + rifapentine x 12 weeks</li><li>rifampin daily x 4 months</li><li>isoniazid daily x 9 months</li></ul>
TB meningitis	–	All 4 first-line drugs together, intensive regimen

Text D

Guiding Parents and Other Caregivers on Vigilance

<u>Direct Observation Therapy (DOT)</u>

Advise caregivers that a healthcare professional will actually watch the child take their TB medicines, either during home visits or video chats (e.g. on phone or computer). This will be an opportunity to exchange information and discuss any side effects.

Emphasise completing the regimen exactly as prescribed, using the supplied measuring device for precise measurements. Interruption of dosing regimen risks emergence of drug resistance and aggravation of illness. Where DOT is not possible, the caregiver should be guided to set an alert for the same time on relevant days.

<u>Contact with Others</u>

Instruct caregivers to monitor others in the household or those with whom the child had close contact prior to treatment. They should note or ask contacts to report:

- coughs that last 3 weeks or more
- swollen glands
- anorexia leading to cachexia
- fever and/or chills
- night sweats

Reassure the adult that the child's condition will usually improve noticeably within a few weeks of starting the drug regimen. After two weeks of taking the medication exactly as prescribed, children are usually no longer contagious and can return to school.

End of Part A | Text booklet

Part B

In this part of the test, there are six short extracts relating to the work of health professionals. For questions **1–6**, choose the answer (**A**, **B** or **C**) that you think fits best according to the text.

Your answers should be made by filling in the circle completely:

1. The memo informs clinicians who are prescribing for HIV patients

    (A) to routinely check the database for new drugs.

    (B) that not all drug interactions must be avoided.

    (C) that the most severe interactions involve prescribed agents.

From: Pharmacy Department
Re: Drug Cautions In HIV
Prescribers must be vigilant regarding drug–drug interactions (DDIs) in patients on antiretroviral therapy (ARV). ARV carries some of the highest DDI risks and can critically affect HIV viral control. Antidepressants, antibiotics and statins are well-recognised dangers, but vitamins and herbal supplements also pose significant risks. Please refer to the online database available to clinicians before prescribing medication to persons taking ARV. The database indicates absolute contraindications as well as relative co-administration alerts, as close monitoring or dose adjustment may be appropriate in some cases.
DDI recommendations are periodically updated as new drugs or new formulations of existing drugs emerge. You may also consult the pharmacy department or HIV specialist for updates.

2. The guidelines state that

    (A) the resuscitation leader is responsible for explaining the active resuscitation process.

    (B) parents must aways be allowed to witness the resuscitation of their child.

    (C) parents can stop or change the resuscitation efforts during the process.

Parental/Authorised Guardian Presence During Pediatric Resuscitation
Hospital policy supports parents and authorised guardians being present during the resuscitation of their children. To ensure that there is no interference with resuscitation and no distraction of the care team, a staff member should always stay with the parents/guardians to explain sympathetically and clearly what is happening. When appropriate and practical, parents/guardians should be allowed physical contact with the child. Space may preclude parents/guardians being close to the bedside during resuscitation efforts. Where possible, observation from outside the room is allowed as long as this does not unduly affect patient privacy and dignity.
The resuscitation team leader should decide when to stop the resuscitation, but parents/guardians may change goals for care while witnessing a resuscitation. This must be documented, including the time and the identity of the authorised parent/guardian making the decision.

3. The main objective of the information is to

   (A) outline the procedure for handling patient belongings.

   (B) provide legal information that both patients and the hospital need.

   (C) to highlight why nurses are responsible for securing patient property.

Handling Of Patient Property
Nurses are responsible for educating patients about securing valuables and about legal disclaimers and limits to hospital responsibility.
Elective admissions should be advised not to bring large amounts of cash or valuables with them, or should arrange for such items to be taken home. Emergency admissions should be evaluated by the medical officer who should document whether the patient is able take responsibility for their belongings.
Lucid patients should hand over relevant valuables to a nurse who should place them in a hospital-provided bag. Sealing of the bag and completion of the Patient Property Duplicate Form must be witnessed by the patient or their guardian, and one copy of the form given to the patient. The bag and form should then be transferred to the Cashier's Office.
For unconscious patients, the hospital has a legal obligation to secure patient property, even without explicit handover.
On loss of patient property, patients and relatives should be advised to seek independent legal advice.

4. The policy statement advises health professionals

   (A) that they may accept all gifts that are under £25.

   (B) that no further action is needed if a gift has been rejected.

   (C) to consider multiple factors when assessing patient motivation for gift-giving.

Hospital Policy: Gifts And Conflicts Of Interest
Accepting gifts may undermine the health professional's integrity, cause conflicts of interest or even raise allegations of bribery. Consider the timing of gifts that may be harmless tokens offered during festive periods or strategically offered ahead of a required medical procedure. Always decline gifts: • of any amount given to secure preferential treatment • that are disproportionately large • that would cause the recipient feelings of discomfort should colleagues know about it • that would clearly or probably cause hardship to the patient's family • of items or vouchers worth more than £25. Declare any gift not accepted, giving the reason why. Where the appropriateness of a gift is not clear, advice from a senior member of staff can be sought.

5. The guidelines make it clear that

   (A) home oxygen concentrators are contraindicated in active smokers.

   (B) patients may be denied home oxygen therapy even if it is strongly indicated clinically.

   (C) home oxygen assessment services may remove LTOT equipment if risk is high.

Prescribing Of Home Oxygen Concentrators
Long-term oxygen therapy (LTOT) is indicated for patients who have repeated acute pulmonary events or persistent blood O2 levels under 92%. In these cases, they and their living situation must be further thoroughly assessed.
Consider patient mental alertness, vision and fall risk, as home oxygen concentrator tubing may pose a hazard and occasional device troubleshooting may be needed. Patients and caregivers should be educated verbally and in writing about keeping the oxygen concentrator at least 6 feet away from pilot lights, flame cookers and lit candles. The risks of home oxygen concentrators in smokers of regular or e-cigarettes should be considered on a case-by-case basis, and those who smoke should be explicitly informed about the dangers of smoking near oxygen and educated about quitting.
Home oxygen assessment services may advise against oxygen concentrator units if they think the risk is too high. Established LTOT may also be discontinued if persistent risks are noted on repeat assessments.

6. Based on the official letter

(A) saying you are sorry after an accident can negatively affect your claim.

(B) you must be seen by a doctor immediately after leaving the accident site.

(C) if an injury was the nurse's fault, he/she must pay for legal advice.

From: National Nursing Association (NNA)

Subject: Accidents At Work

Members of the NNA are eligible for free legal representation if they incur an injury at the workplace which was not their fault. For best representation:

1. report the accident as soon as possible to your nursing supervisor or immediate superior
2. record the incident in your workplace Accident Book
3. be examined as soon as possible by a medical professional who should submit a completed Accident Form to us within 4 days of examining you
4. if possible, take pictures of the accident site and any contributing hazards; note down the serial number of any equipment involved, and obtain contact information from any witnesses.

It is important that you do not apologise or accept responsibility for the incident, even verbally.

Keep records of any resulting sick leave, expenditures related to your treatment and a diary of the treatment itself.

Serious accidents should also be reported to the regional Occupational Safety and Health Agency.

End of Part B

Part C

In this part of the test, there are two texts about different aspects of healthcare. For questions **7–22**, choose the answer (**A**, **B**, **C** or **D**) that you think fits best according to the text.

Your answers should be made by filling in the circle completely: Ⓐ Ⓑ Ⓒ Ⓓ

Text 1: Autism

Scientific understanding of autism has evolved over the last three decades with respect to influences on brain development that play a part in autism development. The timing of first-time diagnoses is occurring earlier in children and much later into adulthood than two decades ago. Greater public awareness and advocacy about autism has laid the groundwork for an increase in the number and extent of services available and, in parallel, expanded expertise and support for persons with autism and for their caregivers. A natural progression from this has been increased debate about definitions and classification of types of autism, and around inclusion of people with autism in education programmes, professions and the community at large.

Estimates of autism prevalence have seen a rapid rise since its redefinition in the 1994 Diagnostic and Statistical Manual IV (DSM-4) along with the increase in overall global population. Prevalence in 2011 was estimated at around 1 in 100 and has since increased, but this does not necessarily mean a real rise in the percentage of those exhibiting features of autism. Changes in definitions and improved screening and diagnostic tools have all played major roles. In 2013, the diagnosis of autism seemingly exploded when autism spectrum disorder (ASD) was declared an umbrella diagnosis covering Asperger's syndrome, autism and other disorders. For the first time, the DSM-5 also allowed the concomitant diagnosis of autism and attention-deficit hyperactivity disorder (ADHD). In 2022, Salari et al. updated global estimates to as many as 1 in 60, but it is important to note that this number should be considered against the background of socio-cultural and economic factors that can affect data collection in each country.

In terms of regional prevalence, differences in definitions, screening tools, research methods and social characteristics must be clarified before strict interpretation of apparent variations between populations. For example, data places ASD prevalence around the Persian Gulf at 0.14–2.9% and in China at 0.2%. This compares to 1.7% in the US and Europe. These apparent disparities may occur when surveys only sample communities that have good access to social services, yielding an underestimation of the true regional number. Cultural differences in how childhood behaviour is perceived might also influence if and when professional assessment is sought. A lack of culture-sensitive diagnostic tools that factor in gender or religion might hinder uptake and impede reliable comparisons between regions. Furthermore, while a standardised tool deployed in-person by a healthcare professional might seem optimal, in reality a clinician could be tempted to over-apply certain labels so as to access study resources that are not routinely available.

ASD diagnosis occurs most often between 2 and 5 years old when developmental milestones in language, play and other behaviours are most noticeable. Those with more severe symptoms are identified earlier because they make no attempt to mimic neurotypical behaviours and communication styles. This early intervention means better opportunities to address functioning. Milder conditions, however, are often missed until very late because the higher level of functionality does encourage **adaptive masking**. Autism having been classified as a pediatric condition up until the 1994 means that potentially high numbers of present-day seniors have missed out on specific information and support for most of their lives because they were either misdiagnosed with anxiety/depression or attention deficit hyperactivity disorder, or because a disorder or comorbidity was not even considered.

Research on contributing factors in ASD has made understanding causation more opaque instead of less. Fragile X syndrome and other genetic variants exist in over one-third of autism cases, while contributing factors in the other two-thirds range from older maternal age and some medications to environmental factors. In 2020, the results of a four-year study by McGuinn et al. found positive associations between ASD risk and exposure to ozone and particulate matter within very specific pre-natal and post-natal time frames. These results bore out data from previous studies. Kang in 2017 found that after microbiome transfer therapy, participants in that study developed not only improved gut bacterial diversity but, compellingly, improved language and social interaction – key issues in autism – and that these changes persisted even at the two-year review. Conversely, fears from the late 1990s of a causal link to the measles-mumps-rubella vaccine or to the preservative, thiomersal, have been proven to be unfounded.

The lack of an exact cause of ASD, however, means that therapies remain reactive rather than proactive. The only scientifically proven yet still-debated autism therapy is applied behavioral analysis (ABA) therapy. ABA therapy identifies specific settings in which functioning is needed and dysfunctions that might occur, and deploys proven behavior modification strategies and reward systems as reinforcement and then re-measures the target behaviour to check for improvement. This may be intense for children with already raised levels of anxiety, and put a strain on caregivers who must participate actively in the process on top of other increased demands. There is also the point that ABA's reward system suggests that there is some implicit negative punishment, even if this is simply the withholding of reward. ABA, however, allows for experimental designs that can manipulate single variables to deliver evidence-based causal links to behavior outcomes, something that is highly regarded by both clinicians and researchers. Speech and language therapy, cognitive behavior therapy, psychotropic drugs and even hyperbaric oxygen are other options that seek to address the range of issues and severities.

There is now debate between those who consider autism a pathology and those who see the spectrum as naturally occurring variations. Those who favour pathology represent a high percentage of caregivers who point out the heavy financial and emotional toll of caring for persons with autism. This group supports ongoing research into neurodevelopment and better and earlier screening tools, and advocates for more to be done for autism diagnosis, including in adults. The other group argues that autism is not a disease to be cured, and pushes for acceptance of neurodiversity in the same way that variations in physical characteristics are accepted, and for accommodation just as those in wheelchairs are accommodated. **It** advocates for more research on social aspects of living with autism. Despite approaching the issue from different sides, both perspectives are united in the common call for more and wider research.

Text 1: Questions 7–14

7. In Paragraph 1, better autism services were noted to be the direct result of

   (A) recognition of earlier stages of the condition.

   (B) scientific understanding of the underlying cause.

   (C) a rise in the number of autism experts 30 years ago.

   (D) general knowledge and demands for more help for autism.

8. Paragraph 2 makes the point that

   (A) rethinking definitions of autism has made it a more common diagnosis.

   (B) too many disorders are now grouped under the autism spectrum diagnosis.

   (C) prevalence of autism would have stayed unchanged without changes in the DSM-5.

   (D) social factors have helped increase the percentage of autism spectrum diagnoses.

9. In Paragraph 3, with regard to ASD prevalence, the author

   (A) highlights how low ASD prevalence is in some regions.

   (B) denies that cultural issues create falsely high ASD estimates.

   (C) emphasises the different roles clinicians have in research.

   (D) demonstrates why available data should not be taken at face value.

10. The term '**adaptive masking**' refers to

    (A) adults being more skilled at hiding symptoms than children.

    (B) the ability to compensate for one behaviour by enhancing another.

    (C) doctors confirming that there is no neurological issue.

    (D) clinicians teaching persons how to modify their severe symptoms.

11. The study by McGuinn et al.

- (A) has become more accepted than other similar studies.
- (B) showed the results of other studies had errors.
- (C) found similar results to other studies done before.
- (D) was not as rigorous as other comparable studies.

12. In Paragraph 6, in terms of ABA therapy, the author

- (A) acknowledges that there are drawbacks to ABA therapy.
- (B) is concerned that there are no proactive therapies.
- (C) is confident other therapies are as effective as ABA.
- (D) is critical of the harsher aspects of ABA.

13. In Paragraph 7, the word '**It**' refers to

- (A) neurodiversity supporters.
- (B) people with autism.
- (C) people in wheelchairs.
- (D) caregivers.

14. The final paragraph makes the point that

- (A) the author strongly supports the pathology perspective.
- (B) the author considers autism in the same light as other disabilities.
- (C) the two sides agree on some aspects of the autism debate.
- (D) there is a stronger push for diagnostic tools for children.

Text 2: One Health

One Health is an approach that acknowledges the link between human health and that of animals, plants and the general ecosystem. It is not a new concept but has become more prominent in the wake of the environmental and microbial changes in recent years. One Health coordinates efforts to address global challenges to health by promoting a sustainable balance to optimise the health of all through purposeful collaboration across different governmental and non-governmental sectors at community, regional, national and global levels. If executed as conceptualised, One Health would tackle issues from prevention to early detection of disease, preparedness for change and response to disaster. Additionally, having a global ideology could, in theory, facilitate understanding of and buy-in to the benefits and trade-offs of sustainable solutions at the crucial individual level within communities. **This** is often where the stumbling block to change occurs, especially in democracies.

One Health covers vector-borne and zoonotic diseases, antimicrobial resistance, food-borne illnesses as well as pollution and climate change. In 2022, the World Bank estimated that implementing the broad One Health approach would cost global economies around $3–4 billion annually but would save over $30 billion annually. This runs counter to the modern attitude of most First World governments with regard to health spending, giving greater focus to disease cures and managing complications. Unarguably, the COVID-19 pandemic highlighted the financial aspect of the interdependency of animal health, the environment and human health, just as the spread of endemic dengue hotspots continues to reflect the link between human health, climate change and disease vectors, and the increase in reactive healthcare spending in temperate-zone First World countries. Accordingly, one World Health Organization (WHO) article used the term '**false economy**' in reference to this contemporary approach.

With a projected 80 million people being added to the world's population each year, estimates put the world's population at roughly 10 billion by 2050. The implementation of One Health will require top-down policies that support national collaboration and strengthen establishment and execution of programmes, as well as technological, structural and organisational changes. Integration of databases must permit more seamless data gathering and sharing, which may challenge national citizens' privacy laws. Human resources will have to be mobilised locally and across borders for routine operations as well as emergency responses. Critically, there must be standardisation of assessments and quality controls, and evaluation of outcomes so that best practice can be shared between countries. This requires involvement not only from the policy makers and the healthcare sector, but also from agriculture, animal husbandry, technology and law enforcement.

It is perhaps an irony that despite the progress made over the last 150 years in the areas of understanding health and developing ill-health cures, the world has reached this juncture. The United Nations 2017 estimate states that by 2050 more than half the world's population will be living even longer and mainly in nine countries covering Asia, Africa and the United States, with over two-thirds of this number concentrated in urban areas. This will amplify issues of food demand, food security and coexisting poverty, especially in the less affluent countries. More attention will be needed to biosecurity, food production and distribution. Higher urban population densities can also increase human-to-human and animal-to-human contact with increased need for sanitation and pest control to prevent zoonotic, vector- and food-borne diseases. Increased crowding also often gives rise to new strains of existing pathogens, as seen with Ebola, H2N1 influenza and severe acute respiratory syndrome (SARS).

The roles of wild and domestic animals and the climate have not been as comprehensively covered as other aspects of One Health. Land and coastal animals are directly impacted by rainfall, drought, flooding and consequent pests and disease. This affects farming practices as well as the finances and food supply of those dependent on these animals. Mitigation of the impacts would require changes to agricultural monitoring systems and practices. Zinsstag et al., 2015, proposed an integrated human and animal surveillance and response model, arguing that it would be significantly more cost-effective if emerging diseases could be detected in vectors, livestock or wildlife before their detection in humans. Traditionally, however, veterinary and public health systems have not been routinely linked.

The fact that One Health so far has no single, internationally adopted definition means there is no rigorous guidance for local drafting and enacting of policies. This has given rise to conflicts in interpretation. Su et al., 2024, noted that although the One Health ideology is holistic, One Health professionals themselves prioritise human life, raising the ethical question of whether crisis management should prioritise human life over that of animals. The significance of this was seen in the public outcries that followed the mass culling of farm animals during COVID-19 and again after the mass culling of EU and UK birds during the 2023 avian flu outbreak, another ethical point related to what constitutes a 'healthy environment'. The value of animals and the environment in One Health is intrinsically framed in the context of their usefulness to humans. Without clear and rigorous guidelines, there will be inevitable varied and convenient interpretations of the term.

There are further challenges to be overcome. The divergent interests and priorities of different regions and sectors can hinder programme timelines and success, just as agencies with different funding and objectives will require significant input and coordination to learn to work together. Collating statistical outcomes from evidence-based research with qualitative information from the environment sector will necessitate the development of new evaluation tools, which will also be needed in areas where there are few objective measurements to monitor. Ultimately, overcoming these hurdles will require countries to invest in resources, meaning that higher-income countries will be better placed to capitalise on One Health benefits than lower income countries, resulting in a consistently widened One Health gap.

15. In Paragraph 1, the author expresses the view that

  A disease screening would receive greater focus under One Health.

  B One Health ideologies are outdated and need revision.

  C the One Health ideology utilises a strategic approach.

  D too frequently, people hinder change for the better.

16. In Paragraph 1, the word '**This**' refers to

  A advantages and disadvantages of solutions.

  B individuals supporting the changes needed.

  C the range of objectives of One Health.

  D having a global ideology about health.

17. In Paragraph 2, the term '**false economy**' is used to reflect

  A too much money being spent on reacting to health disasters.

  B neglecting to invest in preventive public health measures.

  C wrong calculations when costing public health measures.

  D underestimating the annual number of health disasters.

18. The information in Paragraph 3 is given to

  A highlight the problem of the rate of world population growth.

  B explain why technology will be the biggest challenge in One Health.

  C demonstrate how best practice can be achieved.

  D to outline the monumental scope of the One Health undertaking.

19. According to the author in Paragraph 4

- (A) living more in urban areas will contribute to even longer lifespans.
- (B) current and future health challenges are a result of human scientific advancement.
- (C) food distribution may become easier with people concentrated in certain regions.
- (D) improved health will lead to more people moving to urban areas.

20. Zinsstag's 2015 proposal

- (A) misses a crucial element needed to make it viable.
- (B) would be much too expensive to implement.
- (C) would decrease the range of vectors in some areas.
- (D) would reduce strict dependency on animal resources.

21. In Paragraph 6, when considering ethical aspects of One Health, the author is

- (A) in agreement with prioritising human life in decision-making.
- (B) worried more ethical controversies will hinder One Health.
- (C) convinced communities will need externally imposed objective guidelines and definitions.
- (D) impressed that regions are defining One Health for themselves.

22. In the final paragraph, the author makes the point that

- (A) the biggest obstacles are posed by interfaces between sectors.
- (B) poorer countries will remain behind despite One Health's goals.
- (C) merging different data formats is not practical.
- (D) environmental agencies will have to change their research approach.

End of Part C

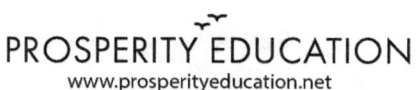

Occupational English Test

Reading

Test 4

Part A

- Look at the four texts (**A–D**) in the accompanying **text booklet**.
- For each question (**1–20**) look through the texts (**A–D**) to find the relevant information.
- Write your answers in the spaces provided in this **question paper**.
- Answer all the questions within the 15-minute time limit.
- Your answers should **only** be taken from texts **A–D** and must be correctly spelt.

Sickle Cell Disease: Questions

Questions 1–7

For each question (**1–7**), decide which text (**A, B, C** or **D**) the information comes from. Write the letter **A, B, C** or **D** in the space provided. You may use any letter more than once.

In which text can you find information about

1   physical problems that occur over time in sickle cell disease (SCD)?   _____

2   protocol for monitoring patients on parenteral opioids?   _____

3   the process doctors should follow when the patient is returning home?   _____

4   how specific parts of the body are affected by SCD?   _____

5   pathogens to be cautious of in SCD?   _____

6   special body fluid tests done in specific situations?   _____

7   who should and should not receive morphine?   _____

Questions 8–14

Answer each of the questions (**8–14**) with a word or short phrase from one of the texts. Each answer may include words, numbers or both. You should **not** write full sentences.

8   What should be measured regularly in patients who receive repeated transfusions?

_____

9   Who should manage patients who call the hospital with non-critical problems?

_____

10 What can happen especially at night when there is chronic kidney impairment?

_____

11 What should be stopped if a patient develops diarrhea and abdominal pain?

_____

12 What body temperature range should trigger transfer of a patient to the ward?

_____

13 What kind of urine culture is done typically in SCD patients?

_____

14 For a pain score of 8, what should be given with the first dose of oral morphine?

_____

Questions 15–20

Complete each of the sentences (**15–20**) with a word or short phrase from one of the texts. Each answer may include words, numbers or both.

15 Patients cleared for discharge should receive _____ along with analgesia.

16 Typically, skeletal X-rays taken just after an acute illness are _____.

17 Vitamin D deficiency is linked to diet and higher _____.

18 The hematology registrar cosigns the patient discharge together with the _____.

19 Parvovirus should be suspected if the proportion of young erythrocytes is less than _____.

20 The lowest body weight that can receive morphine is _____.

End of Part A

Sickle Cell Disease: Texts

Text A

Triage

During normal hours, Monday to Friday: all sickle cell disease (SCD) patients can be assessed and treated on the Hematology Ward.

Otherwise: patients should be immediately directed to Emergency Department (ED).

Non-emergent cases contacting by phone can be dealt with by a triage nurse and, if appropriate, the patient should be guided to present to the hematology ward on the next working day.

Assessment

A thorough history should be taken, noting any life-threatening complications. Examine skin color changes (extreme pallor, cyanosis, jaundice), neurological signs (weakness, lethargy, seizures), and respiratory issues (shortness of breath). Note pain location and score, analgesia previously taken, sites of infection, size of the liver and spleen, and blood pressure.

Immediate ward admission required for

- pain requiring parenteral opioid administration
- shortness of breath and lethargy, especially if examination suggests lung consolidation
- fever of 38C and above, especially with tachycardia and hypotension
- abdominal pain, distension or diarrhea and vomiting
- abnormal CNS signs
- priapism (painful sustained erection >4 hours). Surgical emergency.

Ward discharge

The main care physician should consult the Hematology Registrar on-call for sign off on patient discharge. Confirm that the patient has:

- oral analgesia (NSAIDS, paracetamol), anti-emetics. Laxatives should also be considered as standard
- instructions on daily fluid volume intake
- any required antibiotics (if infection had been confirmed)
- folic acid
- prophylactic penicillin V or erythromycin.

Follow-up appointment within 8 days.

Text B

Routine basic investigations include full blood count, blood group and cross matching, urea, electrolytes and creatinine, liver function tests with lipid screening as a standard, and blood and mid-stream urine cultures for pathogens.

Contingent Investigations

Investigation	Indication
Hb electrophoresis (for % of HbS and HbF)	New patients. HbS done routinely only if patient goes on regular transfusion programme
Capillary or arterial blood gases	Deteriorating O_2 saturations in air
Abdominal ultrasound	Abdominal symptoms/signs; suspected gall bladder complications
Yersinia bacteria screening – stool & serology	In patients • on drug deferoxamine – stop drug if diarrhea and abdominal pain (enterocolitis) develop • with suspected immunocompromise
CT scan of head	Suspected or confirmed neurological complications, including stroke
X-rays of joints, bones, chest*	Bone and joint X-rays – usually unhelpful in acute pain crises CXR – show areas of lung collapse in chest syndromes
ECG	If arrhythmia or angina suspected
Throat, nose, sputum, stool, wound and spinal fluid cultures	Contingent on suspected specific infection
Virus screen (Hepatitis B & C, cytomegalovirus, parvovirus, HIV)	For new patients. Parvovirus testing also done if immature red cell count is under one percent.

X-rays of bones and joints show little or no change in the first six days of a crisis except in cases of avascular necrosis or osteomyelitis.

Text C

Management of Pain Crises

Pain is the most common cause of hospital admission, and needs to be addressed within the first 30 minutes of presentation, with the goal of pain control within 60 minutes. Patient assessment should include information on analgesia taken prior to attending hospital and current pain score.

Unless blood transfusion is needed, general supportive care is given:
- reassurance that pain will soon settle with appropriate analgesia
- keep patient comfortably warm and relaxed
- hydration (oral or IV)
- intravenous access as needed for fluids, analgesia, antibiotics
- identification and treatment of infection
- periodic review of status

Analgesia

Severe pain (score 7–10): In the Emergency Department, give simultaneously intra-nasal diamorphine + first dose of oral morphine. If intranasal route not possible, give oral or bolus IV morphine. Outside of the ED, give either oral or bolus IV morphine. Morphine is contraindicated in:
- <1 year old
- < 10kg weight
- head or nasal injury
- drug sensitivity

Moderate pain (score 4–6): NSAIDs, paracetamol and/or oral morphine as needed

Mild pain (score 1–3): NSAIDs and paracetamol

Monitoring patients on analgesia – done q30min until pain controlled and patient stable then q2h if patient is on IV opioids:
- Pain score
- Sedation level
- Oxygen saturation (room air)
- PR, RR, BP, Temp. If RR falls < 10/minute, discontinue opiate infusion and consider naloxone administration

Text D

Monitoring Ongoing Complications

Life expectancy may be 20 years shorter than average; may be even shorter without prompt interventions.

Short-term:

- Acute pain crises: intense pain due to blocked blood flow in bones and other tissues
- Infections: anemia and a weakened immune system increase risk and frequency of infections
- Acute chest syndrome: caused by obstruction of small vessels in the lung by deformed red cells or fat emboli – results in chest pain, dyspnoea and cyanosis
- Stroke: due to blood vessel blockage in the brain
- Priapism in males – painful sustained erection > 4 hours – surgical emergency

Intermediate and long-term:

- Chronic pain even between acute pain episodes
- Symptomatic anemia due to reduced red cell count
- Organ damage: including to the kidneys, liver and heart. Kidney symptoms include frequency, nocturnal bed-wetting, blood in urine, vomiting, fatigue and hypertension. Liver problems can result in blood sequestration, gallstones, bone necrosis, and leg ulcers. Heart enlargement and failure can occur. Eye problems with sickle retinopathy and retinal detachment. Necrosis of the shoulder and hip joints causing mobility issues.
- Low Vitamin D: due to nutritional intake and increased cell turnover
- Iron overload: may require monthly chelation therapy

End of Part A | Text booklet

Part B

In this part of the test, there are six short extracts relating to the work of health professionals. For questions **1–6**, choose the answer (**A**, **B** or **C**) that you think fits best according to the text.

Your answers should be made by filling in the circle completely: Ⓐ ⬤ Ⓒ

1. What point does the memo make about documenting ulcers present at admission?

    Ⓐ All skin ulcers must be reported using the appropriate forms.

    Ⓑ Skin damage caused by devices should be entered in its own form.

    Ⓒ Only certain ulcers should be detailed on the pressure ulcer form.

To: Nurses
MEMO: Patients With Pressure Ulcers On Admission
On admission, patients who are elderly, mobility-assisted or wearing external devices should be asked about any superficial areas of discomfort or numbness, such as over bony prominences or where a device has direct contact with skin. Patients with decreased sensation due to neurological or other causes may not be aware of early ulcers, and so direct inspection of the skin is required. Nurses should report all pressure ulcers at grade 2 and above that are already present at admission, including details of site, size and grade, supported with photographs, if possible.
Skin damage that is a result of incontinence and/or moisture alone should not be recorded as a pressure ulcer but as moisture-association skin damage.
Skin damage due to a device, such as casts or ventilator tubing and masks, must be similarly documented as device-related pressure ulcers.

2. What do the guidelines say about wrongful resuscitation due to a missed DNR order?

   (A) The main clinician should hand over to another clinical team.

   (B) All medical measures should stop once the DNR is noted.

   (C) Administration of palliative care should continue.

Do Not Resuscitate Protocol (DNR)
When the DNR protocol is activated, clinicians should conduct an initial assessment, perform basic medical care including: clearing and suctioning of the airway, administering oxygen, and maintain any IV access for hydration or medication to relieve discomfort only but not to prolong life. Clinicians should not perform CPR, insert artificial airways, defibrillate, cardio convert or do continuous cardiac monitoring.
Should the clinician or team administrating resuscitation only be made aware of the DNR after resuscitation has begun, all non-basic care activities must then cease and the events documented in the patient records.
Main care clinicians who are unwilling or unable to comply with the DNR order must still administer basic medical care and not delay in handing over to another clinician who will carry out the DNR protocol.

3. The main purpose of the information is to

   (A) outline the principal issues to be checked during a heatwave.

   (B) identify patients who are at highest risk during a heatwave.

   (C) describe how to create cooler room temperatures for patients.

Patients' Care During Heatwaves
Record indoor temperatures regularly and keep rooms or areas below 26°C, if possible. Use shades or cover windows and turn off unnecessary lights or equipment. Identify specific 'cool rooms' that can be used for high-risk scenarios.
Prioritise those patients most vulnerable to heat sickness (e.g. >65 years old, infection, kidney and cardiovascular problems). If moving high-risk patients to a cooler room is not feasible or possible, use alternative strategies to cool them (e.g. extra liquids, cool wipes). Increase monitoring of vitals and urine input-output. Consider weighing vulnerable patients to detect early dehydration and consider adjusting bedding and clothing. Discharge planning should take home temperatures and the available support into account.
Most medicines should be stored below 25°C, out of direct sunlight and in a dry area. Consult Pharmacy Services for further guidance on storage of specific medications.

4. What does the instruction manual imply about weighing patients accurately?

   (A) A list of the fixed-weight additional bed items should be kept.

   (B) Too many items in the bed increases the chances of inaccuracy.

   (C) All items should be removed from the bed during patient weighing.

Using Smart Bed Features To Weigh Patients
The Patient Scale has a 1% margin of error, with most accurate weights achieved when the bed is not touching anything including walls, machines affixed to walls or fillable-drainage containers.
Before placing a new patient on the bed, the sleep surface must be prepared by weighing the bed with all pillows, blankets and other fixed-weight items that the patient will be using while on the bed. If the patient is to be transferred to and from the bed, check to ensure fixed-weight items remain constant.
During weighing operation, the bed should be between horizontal and head-position 40 degrees below the horizontal, with most accurate readings seen between 30 to 40 degrees. No one should touch the bed when the scale is operating.

5. The policy document informs staff that they

   (A) may use mobile phones for personal use during emergency situations.

   (B) may use their phone's verbal command features during official breaks.

   (C) are not permitted to access social media during work hours when in the hospital.

POLICY DOCUMENT: Use Of Personal Mobile Phones At Work
Mobile phones, headphones and airbuds should be out of sight in patient-care settings but may be placed in silent or silent-vibrate mode. Voice-activated speaker features are prohibited during patient care. All mobile device use is prohibited during medication preparation and disbursement to avoid distraction. Mobile devices must not be used for accessing social media or video-streaming sites unless pre-approved by the Administration Office. Personal mobile-device use is limited to official break times either within designated break rooms or off hospital grounds. Mobile devices are part of this hospital's emergency plan. When the emergency protocol is activated, mobile-device use is allowed for direct patient care through the secure hospital app. These policies apply to situations where employees are in view or outside of view of patients and/or visitors.

6. What point does the correspondence make about documentation in domestic-abuse cases?

    (A) Patients must give consent for any domestic-abuse screening.

    (B) Any healthcare staff professional can prepare reports for abuse lawsuits.

    (C) Clinicians can document domestic abuse even when it is not confirmed.

| **To: Clinicians** |
| **TOPIC: Documentation For Domestic Abuse In Adults** |
| It may not be possible to elicit sensitive information from patients who are suspected abuse victims, and there may be explicit denial by the patient. Nurses and doctors are mandated abuse reporters, nonetheless, and have a duty of care to document the patient's appearance and behaviour using non-judgmental language. Responses to screening questions and any disclosures about abuse should be entered using the patient's own words, as far as possible. Physical injuries can be photographed with permission.

Patients may require letters or reports in support of abuse, either for litigation or legal-aid applications. Letters and reports can be provided by a doctor, nurse, midwife, psychologist or health visitor. |

End of Part B

Part C

In this part of the test, there are two texts about different aspects of healthcare. For questions **7–22**, choose the answer (**A**, **B**, **C** or **D**) that you think fits best according to the text.

Your answers should be made by filling in the circle completely: Ⓐ Ⓑ Ⓒ Ⓓ

Text 1: Gene Therapy

Gene therapy (GT) is a cutting-edge approach that offers treatment for some disorders that previously had none. Inserting new copies of a gene into cells, altering sections of the genome or blocking genes from creating malfunctioning proteins can relieve symptoms or cure disease. What is more, GT techniques can, in theory, be applied to reproductive cells to prevent or augment the transfer of genes, and therefore characteristics, to offspring. As of 2023, there were more than 100 gene therapies approved for use worldwide. Some cancers, blood disorders, eye diseases and HIV/AIDS are already treatable with GT, and the list is growing. This groundbreaking capability inevitably raises expected and legitimate questions about risks, use, accessibility and the powerful safeguards needed.

Patient safety is paramount. Herpes, adeno and retroviruses are frequently used as vectors for the insertion of materials into human cells thanks to their unique abilities in entering cells. Scientists exploit this ability by deactivating the virus and using it to deliver a spliced **therapeutic cargo** into human cells. But once in place, there is the risk of virus dormancy with later reactivation and infection, or there may be unpredicted side effects that increase risk of later malignancy. These scenarios mean that there must be a commitment to long-term and intensive patient monitoring.

Sex cell manipulation to silence genes in future offspring can have unintended consequences in other parts of the child's genome. Successful gene silencing could ostensibly encourage eugenics, the engineering of 'ideal' characteristics into human populations, with potential future disenfranchisement of those lacking these characteristics. Yet, it is an irrefutable fact that discovery in the early 2000s of the role of the so-named CRISPR family of DNA sequences, which allows bacteria to identify harmful DNA sequences in invading viruses and create enzymes to destroy the virus, has had far-reaching implications for defeating a number of deadly human cancers and infections through its use in manipulating somatic cells.

Current expectations amongst recipient populations may not match reality, however. GT is still largely experimental, and a 2020 systematic review of research into public and patient perceptions led by Aiyegbusi found widespread confusion and unrealistic expectations about the goals of trial phases, including initial trials to establish safety as well as phases designed to tackle therapeutic benefits. The mainstream media's focus on the more dramatic aspects of GT likely contribute to widespread misperceptions, and **this** will need to be strategically managed or countered to safeguard continuing public support for GT development. Stakeholders, including the public, need a realistic view of its current status, limitations and future prospects.

An idealistic view also emerging from the aforementioned systematic review was that US$1,000 was reasonable for a course of GT, a very far cry from reality. In 2023, the UK, US, Saudi Arabia and Bahrain approved the therapy Casgevy for the treatment of sickle cell disease, a devastating blood disorder affecting 8 million people worldwide and causing 400,000 annual deaths. Casgevy costs U$2.2 million per patient, which limits accessibility to only governments, the wealthy or patients sponsored by the wealthy. This is typical of current therapies, risking their withdrawal from the market, not due to a lack of need but to a lack of sustainable affordability. For-profit pharmaceutical companies fund treatment development, and recouping financial investment is their priority. It is hoped that in time we will see improvements in manufacturing logistics and technology, thereby lowering GT prices to within reach of a larger percentage of those who actually need it.

GT trial participants at present may not ideally represent the target population, and this increases risk when a therapy is finally approved for use. 80% of people living with sickle cell disease live in Sub-Saharan Africa and India, yet clinical trials for sickle cell GT were conducted in the US, Canada and Europe. Additionally, regulatory guidelines meant that trial participants were over 12 years old when the overall global preponderance of sickle cell disease is among children. This missed opportunity to conduct trial therapies in the very populations where they would be most taken up prevented the therapy from becoming more affordable, even in wealthier countries. The highest percentage of sickle cell disease is found in low- and middle-income countries, locations that could facilitate lower development, logistical and production costs. Equitable partnering with these countries could provide global benefits.

Entities developing gene therapies must navigate a complex obstacle course of intellectual property patents related to vectors and technologies. This escalates cost and time, and restricts the number of developers entering the field. These constraints could be partly mitigated if more developers collaborated, agreed to mutually license and use open-source models at stages where it is appropriate. Where patent ownership causes repeated delays, government incentives could help with the transfer of technology, including to regions where the disease is prevalent. Governments of these regions would likely be motivated to address diseases that hit their populations more severely.

GT changes the landscape even at the level of community general practitioners who must now know whether a patient has had GT and which products, as it may impact even their response to antibiotics, steroids, analgesics and even over-the-counter supplements. Beyond health and nutrition, in athletics there are already steps being taken to develop tests to detect GT technology for instances of illicit 'gene doping' at elite levels of sports. Perhaps the next natural evolution in GT will not only be eugenics, but bespoke patient therapy as a norm.

Text 1: Questions 7–14

7. In Paragraph 1, the author is

    (A) surprised at the number of illnesses where gene therapy can be used.

    (B) pragmatic about the range of concerns being raised.

    (C) worried that intensive monitoring will hinder GT progress.

    (D) pleased that the full potential of GT is being explored.

8. The term '**therapeutic cargo**' refers to

    (A) the kind of virus used in vector gene therapy.

    (B) the reprogrammed virus that is injected into the patient.

    (C) the reactivation of the virus after the dormant period.

    (D) corrective material that has been attached to the vector.

9. What main point does the author make in Paragraph 3?

    (A) Children may be most negatively affected by GT.

    (B) The hazards of GT are less persuasive than their benefits.

    (C) Certain GT techniques must be improved to lessen their risk.

    (D) Using GT to improve future humans is fundamentally wrong.

10. In Paragraph 4, the word '**this**' refers to

    (A) Aiyegbusi's systematic review.

    (B) confusion about safety trials.

    (C) what the media highlights.

    (D) misunderstanding about therapeutic benefit.

11. The example of Casgevy in Paragraph 5 is given to show

- (A) how a highly effective drug can fail to help patients.
- (B) which countries are leading the way in routinising GT.
- (C) the kinds of disorders that GT addresses.
- (D) a tactic drug companies use to increase profits.

12. What aspect of the clinical trials does the author criticise in Paragraph 6?

- (A) That the therapy is only approved in certain countries
- (B) The way the trials were designed.
- (C) The limited number of adult trial participants.
- (D) The variation in regulatory guidelines for clinical trials.

13. In Paragraph 7, one way suggested to overcome patent obstacles is to

- (A) move all processes to another country.
- (B) transfer licenses to partner developers.
- (C) use public domain processes.
- (D) encourage more developers to join the sector.

14. What does the author suggest about the future in the final paragraph?

- (A) People may receive GT made specifically for them.
- (B) General practitioners will be able to administer GT.
- (C) Athletes may legitimately access GT in training.
- (D) The risk of drug interactions with GT is expected to decrease.

Text 2: Body Mass index

In the 1930s, Belgian mathematician Adolphe Quetelet developed a calculation to assist in defining the 'average man' among European males by using the simple formula of weight divided by height in meters squared. Forty years later, American physiologist Ancel Keys sought a simple tool for large-scale epidemiological studies on obesity and heart disease, and rebranded the formula as the body mass index (BMI), leading to its wide adoption, including within medical contexts. This genesis of BMI would arguably not meet modern standards for research precision. Mass is a function of density and volume, not height, as in Quetelet's formula. Furthermore, Quetelet's study population was comprised only of western-European men, which raises questions about reproducibility of results in other populations. **These** form the starting points of criticisms by modern healthcare professionals who state that BMI is over-valued as a modern health indicator.

An objective index is required to track obesity and co-morbidities over time within populations and across studies, and the BMI has undergone a plethora of studies. A 2016 meta-analysis by the Global BMI Mortality Collaboration, covering 10 million persons in 239 studies across Asia, Australia, Europe and North America, found that across all study regions, BMI-defined overweight and obesity were statistically associated with higher mortality from all causes including coronary heart disease, stroke and cancer. This suggests that BMI is in fact a tangible basis for tackling obesity at the population level, but this might not automatically translate into viable use for individual patients.

Modern research shows variation in healthy weight ranges between ethnicities: what is healthy for Polynesians differs from that for Asians. Bodies carry weight differently throughout their lifetimes, with the weakest fat-to-BMI correlation in 50–59-year-old women of Korean, Mexican and African descent. BMI also does not differentiate lean from fat mass nor patterns of fat distribution, important because fat around the waist is linked to higher disease risk than fat elsewhere. Despite these facts, the Centre for Disease Control, the National Institute of Health and other global institutions promote the BMI for defining health status, albeit by urging its use together with other health indices such as blood pressure, glucose and cholesterol levels. But many practitioners call for its total abolition.

There are those who are metabolically healthy while being defined by BMI as overweight or obese. Conversely, BMI can be in the healthy range in the presence of metabolic disease. Over-emphasising BMI in heavier persons risks clinicians attributing symptoms mostly or entirely to weight, delaying exploration of other causes or missing diagnoses altogether. In some settings, BMI is recorded in up to 96% of patients' routine health checks, even when the data has no relevance to the patient's care, and despite a lack of evidence that doing so affords measurable benefits to patient care, morbidity or mortality. This raises the question of why such data is being routinely collected.

A well-documented case of a patient with autoimmune disease and high muscle mass attests to the caution needed in applying BMI. Female B had been experiencing persistent health issues despite a relatively healthy lifestyle. With a BMI of 31 classifying her as obese, she was guided to undergo an arduous weight-loss programme until investigation by a second doctor revealed the true cause of her symptoms. Belatedly, she was started on the correct treatment, but by then had endured significant physical and emotional stress and worsening of disease. Where BMI serves as the basis for disqualifying or qualifying patients for investigations, procedures or participation in clinical trials, extreme prudence is also needed to avoid erosion of patient trust.

Obesity was officially recognised as a disease by the National Institute of Health in 1998. Today, fitness coaches, nutritionists, educational institutions and employers have embraced and integrated the BMI. Compared to other fat-assessment methods, such as bio-electrical impedance, underwater weighing, and CT or MRI scans, BMI is simple, immediate, cheap and noninvasive. But individuals risk finding themselves on yet another **slippery slope** of being diagnosed with a recognised disease without having seen a doctor. A high BMI, regardless of physical characteristics, can automatically increase health insurance premiums up to 50% over premiums assigned by so-called 'healthy' BMI values, imposing a financial burden on patients who can often least afford it, and leading to reduction or rejection of coverage for those who may be most in need.

Skinfold thickness is an alternative to BMI, but reliability depends on correct use of the skinfold caliper, and measurement of skin elasticity and hydration level. Waist-to-hip ratio (WHR) matches the simplicity of BMI, with precisely defined zones to be measured. A healthy WHR is 0.9 or less for men and 0.85 or less for women, and its recommended use is supported by research. Two independent 2011 studies by Chernichow et al. and Srikanthan et al. showed that WHR is a more positive linear predictor of obesity-related risk for mortality from all causes. A definite relationship between BMI, mortality risk and mortality cause also exists but is less mathematically consistent even within the same demographic.

There is a need for an accurate, practical and affordable tool to reliably define obesity in a wide range of body types, describe current patient health and predict morbidity and mortality risk at population as well as individual levels. An ideal tool would also not marginalise or worsen healthcare disparities for any group. This presents a distinct challenge. Funding considerations and the cementing of BMI into current practice hinders more rapid progress in this area. The solution may rest, not in developing a new index, but in the algorithmic manipulation of existing tools, requiring researchers to once again call on mathematicians for help.

15. In Paragraph 1, '**These**' refers to

- (A) the demographic used in original study.
- (B) the numbers used in Quetelet's calculation.
- (C) errors in the data Quetelet used.
- (D) modern healthcare professionals.

16. In Paragraph 2, the author makes the point that BMI

- (A) satisfies all requirements as a health indicator.
- (B) value is proven and requires no further evidence.
- (C) is best for tracking obesity and heart disease.
- (D) shows definite validity for a specific parameter.

17. The purpose of Paragraph 3 is to

- (A) show why BMI should not be used in certain groups.
- (B) demonstrate why major organisations still encourage its use.
- (C) emphasise shortcomings in the calculation of BMI.
- (D) highlight its use with other health parameters.

18. In Paragraph 4, when discussing collection of BMI data, the author suggests that

- (A) weight data should be recorded at every patient visit.
- (B) doctors should not consider BMI except in metabolic disease.
- (C) BMI will be incorrectly calculated in some patients.
- (D) BMI documentation might be out of habit rather than need.

19. In Paragraph 5, the author uses the example of Patient B to demonstrate

- (A) why BMI alone should not be the basis for treatment.
- (B) why the patient's BMI should not have been recorded.
- (C) how an incorrect BMI calculation can lead to incorrect treatment.
- (D) an example of a patient incorrectly disqualified from a treatment.

20. The term '**slippery slope**' refers to

- (A) having more symptoms attributed to excess weight.
- (B) facing potential difficulties after receiving unqualified health assessments.
- (C) having more clinicians make the same diagnosis.
- (D) spending more money for diagnosis and treatment.

21. What point does the author make about waist-to-hip ratio (WHR) in Paragraph 7?

- (A) It requires more technical skill to calculate than BMI.
- (B) It is a more robust health indicator than BMI.
- (C) It can be calculated more accurately than BMI in some demographics.
- (D) It does not define clearly when someone is obese.

22. In the final paragraph, the author proposes that in improving on the BMI

- (A) healthcare should seek help from outside the sector.
- (B) any tool that excludes certain groups is unacceptable.
- (C) no single tool can perform all the functions needed.
- (D) stakeholders must work harder to secure research funding.

End of Part C

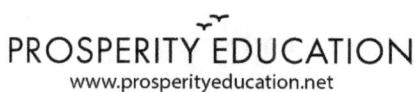

Occupational English Test

Reading

Test 5

Part A

- Look at the four texts (**A–D**) in the accompanying **text booklet**.
- For each question (**1–20**) look through the texts (**A–D**) to find the relevant information.
- Write your answers in the spaces provided in this **question paper**.
- Answer all the questions within the 15-minute time limit.
- Your answers should **only** be taken from texts **A–D** and must be correctly spelt.

Acne: Questions

Questions 1–7

For each question (**1–7**), decide which text (**A, B, C** or **D**) the information comes from. Write the letter **A, B, C** or **D** in the space provided. You may use any letter more than once.

In which text can you find information about

1. non-physical problems that can occur in acne? _____

2. skeletal joint symptoms that occur in a specific kind of acne? _____

3. kinds of surgical interventions used for acne? _____

4. what causes acne lesions to form? _____

5. mechanism of action of different acne treatments? _____

6. complications that medications might cause? _____

7. quantities of formulations to be taken by mouth? _____

Questions 8–14

Answer each of the questions (**8–14**) with a word or short phrase from one of the texts. Each answer may include words, numbers or both. You should **not** write full sentences.

8. What kind of treatment is not indicated in acne fulminans?

   _____

9. In acne conglobata, what is found between skin lesions?

   _____

10 What is the strength of the preferred antibiotic used externally on the skin?

_____

11 What is the shortest recommended time between isotretinoin regimens?

_____

12 In lesions that are not open, what cannot be easily ejected?

_____

13 Which organs are larger in size than normal in acne fulminans?

_____

14 What kind of injections may skin specialists need to administer for cystic acne?

_____

Questions 15–20

Complete each of the sentences (**15–20**) with a word or short phrase from one of the texts. Each answer may include words, numbers or both.

15 Patients should not consume _____ at the same time they take azithromycin.

16 In women, growths that are _____ can cause acne.

17 Referral in acne fulminans should be on an _____ basis.

18 The pattern of fever in acne fulminans is _____.

19 One surgical procedure that must be redone at regular intervals is _____.

20 In women whose lesions are not severe, _____ is an alternative to antibiotics or oral contraceptives.

End of Part A

Acne: Texts

Text A

Overview

Acne vulgaris, the most frequent acne form found on face and trunk, occurs during puberty, pregnancy or with endocrine abnormalities such as virilising tumors in females. Follicles become blocked by excess sebum, cells and, sometimes, inflammation.

Sebum impaction inside follicles creates comedones, which can be non-inflammatory and are either closed by skin cells or open at the skin surface. In closed comedones, keratinised plugs cannot be easily extruded, increasing the chance of inflammation.

Cutibacterium acnes in closed comedones converts sebum into fatty acids, causing irritation within hair follicles. This attracts white blood cells that damage the follicular epithelium and can rupture into the surrounding dermis to form papules and pustules.

Mild acne	<20 comedones OR <15 inflammatory lesions OR <30 total lesions
Moderate acne	20–100 comedones OR 15–50 inflammatory lesions OR 30–125 total lesions
Severe acne	>5 cysts OR >50 inflammatory lesions OR >125 total lesions

Topical monotherapy is typical in acne vulgaris, and maintenance in more severe forms:

- Retinoid gels: increase cell turnover and decrease inflammation
- Benzyl peroxide: bactericidal and reduces excess sebum production
- Clindamycin gel 1%: effective first-line antibiotic
- Clascoterone: anti-androgen; decreases sebum
- Salicylic and azelaic acids: anti-inflammatory and exfoliant' loosen dead cells to prevent clogging

Acne usually settles naturally or with the correction of the underlying disorder. Complicated forms require further specialist referral.

Text B

Oral Regimens

Topical therapies can be continued simultaneously. Oral drugs should be tapered to the lowest maintenance dose once control achieved. Long-term antibiotics may cause a peri-nasal folliculitis, treatable with oral isotretinoin or ampicillin.

	Drug	Duration	Dose	Adverse Reactions & Cautions
Moderate acne*	Doxycycline OR Minocycline	2–3 months	50–100mg twice daily Taken with food	Doxycycline – skin photosensitivity Minocycline – drug-induced lupus and hyperpigmentation (with chronic use)
	Tetracycline	3–4 months	500mg twice daily Not to be taken with food	Skin photosensitivity, gastric upset, fungal infections Taken in 2nd or 3rd trimester; can lead to discoloration in baby's emerging teeth.
	Erythromycin	6–8 weeks; maximum 6 months	500mg twice daily	Gastric upset Increased risk of antibiotic resistance
	Azithromycin	Maximum 3 months	500mg daily, 3 days per week Not to be taken with antacids	Jaundice, abdominal pains Increased risk of antibiotic resistance Rare anaphylactic reaction
Severe acne	Isotretinoin	4–5 months	Start with 1 mg/kg; increase to 2 mg/kg once daily Minimum 0.5 mg/kg daily if side effects extreme	Mucosal dryness, joint pain, depression Absolute contraindication: one month pre-conception, during pregnancy, and one month post-natal Minimum of 4 months between first and follow-up course

*In females with moderate acne who are unresponsive to oral antibiotics, a trial of oral contraceptives or spironolactone may be considered.

Text C

Referral Guidelines

Referral to a specialist is recommended for the following clinical features:

Dermatologist
- Moderate acne not responding to two complete courses of treatment
- Small scars appropriate for chemical peel or dermabrasion
- Cystic acne requiring intralesional injection
- Severe acne variants and similar presentations:
    - Pyoderma faciale – with rapid severe onset, almost exclusively in women 20–50 years old, but does not start with comedones
    - Acne conglobata – with deep cysts and inflamed abscesses commonly joined by sinus tracts causing significant disfigurement
    - Acne fulminans – severe cysts and nodules in adolescent males who also exhibit fever and myalgia. Requires urgent review by an internist.

Internist
- Suspected underlying endocrine disorder (e.g. polycystic ovarian syndrome, adrenal tumors)
- Acne fulminans

Plastic surgeon
- Wide, shallow depressions treatable with injection of fillers. Patients should be advised that fillers (e.g. collagen, hyaluronic acid, polymethylmethacrylate) have temporary effect and must be repeated periodically.
- Deeper scars for excision

Counseling

It is important to treat not only the lesions but also any associated psychological distress, such as:
- being/feeling bullied
- anxiety/depression
- social withdrawal / deteriorating personal relationships
- negative body image

Text D

Acne Fulminans

Clinical features

Acne fulminans is a rare but severe form of acne vulgaris that overwhelmingly affects adolescent males 13–23 years old. It is linked to increased androgens and autoimmune reactions to *Cutibacterium acnes*, a normal skin bacterium. There may be a familial tendency. It can also be triggered by taking anabolic steroids or oral isotretinoin. Onset is abrupt with nodules and cysts 5mm or greater in diameter, ulceration on the chest and back, fluctuating fever, pain in the sacroiliac joints and large joints of the limbs, malaise, anorexia and weight loss. The liver and spleen are frequently enlarged.

Test profile

- Low haemoglobin
- Raised leukocyte count
- Raised erythrocyte sedimentation rate and C-reactive protein (markers of inflammation)
- High male hormones (dehydroepiandrosterone sulfate (DHEAS) and testosterone)
- X-rays show osteolytic lesions

Treatment

- Systemic corticosteroids – prednisone 0.5–1 mg/kg/day for 6 weeks in a tapering dose
- Anti-inflammatory medications (e.g. aspirin)
- Dapsone 50–100 mg/day
- Cyclosporine 5 mg/kg/day
- Oral erythromycin 2 g/day to treat for secondary infection
- Isotretinoin – low dose if not implicated as cause of the eruption
- Tumour Necrosis Factor-alpha inhibitors (e.g. infliximab)
- Unlike most forms of acne vulgaris, topical acne treatments are not helpful in acne fulminans

End of Part A | Text booklet

Part B

In this part of the test, there are six short extracts relating to the work of health professionals. For questions **1–6**, choose the answer (**A, B** or **C**) that you think fits best according to the text.

Your answers should be made by filling in the circle completely: Ⓐ ⬤ Ⓒ

1. According to the text, the health insurer

   A   does not have to pre-approve all out-of-network referrals.

   B   can influence the timing of the referral appointment.

   C   cannot withdraw consent for within-network referrals.

Specialist Referrals Within The Managed Care Network
A 'Managed Care Network' is the group of organisational healthcare services that a patient may access for care covered under their defined health insurance service.
Once referral is being considered, check if the clinician or facility participates fully or conditionally in your patient's insurance plan. If they are outside their managed-care network's plan, your patient may accept to pay privately out of pocket. Your patient should clearly understand why the referral is pertinent to their management, including options, benefits and risks. Ultimately, it is up to them to decide to proceed with the referral, and you should document whether your facility or the patient will make the actual appointment.
Some referrals within a network plan may still require prior approval from the health insurer. It might be possible to avoid referrals by contacting the specialist or facility by phone or tele-meeting to obtain guidance to help you deliver the needed care.

2. The information tells nurses to guide patients on

   (A) a particular directional hair-removal technique.

   (B) the importance of never using soaps to clean the ostomy area.

   (C) rinsing with water at a specific temperature.

To: Nurses

Topic: Guiding Patients On Stoma Bag Skin Care

Patients should be instructed to use warm water to clean around the ostomy, avoiding routine use of soap or baby wipes, as these can leave residues that cause skin inflammation or hamper ostomy-bag adhesion. If soap must be used, it should not contain oils, and the skin should be rinsed well with plain water. For patients insisting on cleansing products, emphasis should be placed on those specifically manufactured for peristomal skin care.

Shaving hairy skin in the area of the ostomy bag can prevent irritation. Electric shavers are recommended but if patients opt for simple safety razors, they should be instructed on shaving away from the stoma in an outward motion, the addition of a wet lubricant and thorough skin-drying after shaving.

3. What guidance does the text give about securing accurate blood glucose results?

   (A) Insulin levels in the days before the test should have been stable.

   (B) Medically prescribed bed rest prior to testing could invalidate glucose results.

   (C) Testing samples at or near to the blood-taking location can help accuracy.

Avoiding Inaccuracies In Blood Glucose Testing
When performing a full 75g oral glucose tolerance test, care must be taken in order to ensure accurate, reflective blood glucose values.
Eating, drinking and routine activity should have been normal in the three days prior to the test.
On the morning of the test, the fasted patient should not have fever, vomiting, parenteral drugs affecting insulin activity (e.g. L-thyroxine, progesterone, glucocorticoids) or gastrointestinal malabsorption, including that from upper GI surgery.
Whole-venous blood collection and testing should follow the guidelines provided by the collection container manufacturer. Containers should be within the expiry date, without signs of damage or tampering, and contain an appropriate anticoagulant. If being transported to a secondary site, sufficient glycolysis-inhibiting agent should also be present. Inadequate inhibition of glycolysis is the most common reason for inaccuracies.

4. The main aim of the appendix is to highlight

   (A) that staff on strike will not get full salary.

   (B) which workers can and cannot go on strike.

   (C) the rules governing how and when strikes occur.

Appendix: Industrial Action By Nurses

Official industrial action must comply with legislation and Nursing Association Guidelines, and be endorsed by a recognised trade union, which in turn must give the employer written notice at least seven days in advance of any action. Industrial action should ensue only after a failure of negotiations, and may be curtailed by the introduction of mediation, concessions or a judgement.

Nurses may legally participate in industrial action as long as essential services continue, and they will not be paid for the strike period. Staff excluded from participating in industrial action are those who provide emergency interventions that directly save lives or prevent potential disability, or who carry out procedures that give information on life-threatening conditions or conditions that can cause permanent disability.

5. According to the guidance for pharmacists, in case of a drug recall, they

- (A) should prioritise recalls announced in the news or online.
- (B) should educate the patient about different drugs with similar effects.
- (C) can advise an affected patient to continue taking the recalled drug.

MEMO: Pharmacists' Duty In Drug Recalls
Pharmacists must be acquainted with the official drug advisory body's (DAB) drug-recall process. Public notification via the DAB website or news media is typical only if a recalled product has been extensively distributed or poses a serious health hazard. However, all recalls, including those for benign reasons such as minor labelling errors, are listed in the DAB's weekly report, and this information should be compared with patients' prescriptions. Cessation of a patient's specific prescription may not be necessary if a particular lot is proven not to be affected or if recall is for benign reasons, not involving issues of drug composition, efficacy or safety, and where no injury has been reported.
Affected patients should not abruptly stop their medication but be guided to either continue with a replacement from an unaffected lot or from a different manufacturer, if feasible, or to contact their doctor with queries about appropriate alternative therapy.

6. The memo argues that the two patients who experienced complications with PCA

   (A) should not have been given the single analgesia starter dose.

   (B) had similar diagnoses and higher-than-recommended drug doses.

   (C) had sleep apnea diagnoses that had been missed during assessment.

MEMO: Patient-controlled Analgesia In Obese Patients With Obstructive Sleep Apnoea
Concerns have been raised about post-operative patients with morbid obesity receiving patient-controlled analgesia (PCA) following two cases of respiratory depression within this group. The patients involved were noted to have had suspected obstructive sleep apnea in addition to PCA equipment which delivered both a background infusion and patient on-demand doses.
Literature shows that PCA without a background infusion has been used safely and effectively for pain relief in morbidly obese patients. However, background infusions should be disabled in any patient with confirmed sleep apnea. Post-operative patients with morbid obesity and suspected sleep apnea should have more intensive monitoring of PCA, judicious background infusions, and a smaller initial bolus dose of analgesia.

End of Part B

Part C

In this part of the test, there are two texts about different aspects of healthcare. For questions **7–22**, choose the answer (**A**, **B**, **C** or **D**) that you think fits best according to the text.

Your answers should be made by filling in the circle completely:

Text 1: Music Therapy in Dementia

50 million people globally have dementia, with a projected doubling of this number by 2050. Pharmaceuticals remain the first line for treating the deterioration in memory, execution, language and social cognition, as well as the depression and anxiety that are common, but **these** are limited in their impact on alleviating attention, interpersonal and other behavioural symptoms. Among non-pharmaceuticals, music is emerging as one of the complementary therapies generating increasing interest. It has been shown to positively impact behavioral disturbances in dementia patients. There have been claims of music effecting pain reduction and improved cognition, but there is much inconsistency in results concerning the strength and reproducibility of the impacts.

The brain processes music through multiple specialised areas, but music is additionally able to bypass the basal ganglia that normally play a role in movement, learning and emotions, and which degenerate in disorders such as dementia and Parkinson's. This rerouting is of no small significance for practical dementia care, as music can stimulate neuronal connections in other areas of the brain that may lose function due to the typical increased apathy that occurs over time. Multiple early studies also reported improved verbal fluency after music therapy, even in those who have largely lost verbal communication skills, suggesting the persistence of a co-existing, alternative route to language production.

A 2014 German study by Keeler et al. further showed that compared to simple conversation, group-singing markedly increased the brain's production of oxytocin, the so-called 'cuddle hormone'. Music production also increases dopamine, the 'reward hormone', even more than simple passive listening. In Alzheimer's, which accounts for 60–70% of dementia cases, age-related dopamine loss parallels cognitive decline, begging the question of whether stimulating dopamine release through music production might help to prevent or slow age-related cognitive decline. This idea is further encouraged by studies showing that not only do musicians tend to have a brain age younger than their chronological age, but they also have lower incidences of dementia.

The many music therapy studies published to date have yielded inconsistent results, however. Until 2020, studies generally focused on improvements in cognitive, emotional, behavioral and psychological symptoms seen with music therapy. More meta-analyses conducted since 2020 have noted no statistically significant impact on dementia-related depression, overall cognition, agitation and daily functioning. Most recently, a UK psychiatric ward using professional music therapists reported a marked reduction in disruptive behaviours among patients on music-therapy days. Meanwhile the first multinational music therapy intervention study, HOMESIDE, running from 2019–2022, focused on music therapy provided by family caregivers in the home setting and showed no longer-term improvements in psychological symptoms beyond the actual engagement with the music. This array of small-study sizes, together with the non-standardised music therapies, lack of dementia classification within samples and absence of longitudinal studies of long-term effects mean that understanding what constitutes best practice remains **a faint light on the horizon**.

The HOMESIDE study also touched on the lesser-highlighted but equally important impact on the family caregiver. In most countries, family members carry a large burden of homecare for dementia patients. HOMESIDE found that caregivers who fully participated in singing therapy with their relatives experienced their own improvements in resilience, and felt that it enhanced the communication and relationship with their relative. This has significant implications for ongoing community support and advice. For example, more than the three professional training sessions offered in this study could be given, with at least one being in-home supervision, especially in situations where financial and family resources are limited and residential placement is not possible.

Music therapy is not without risk in the hands of a well-intentioned but initially ill-equipped caregiver. Music intervention may need to be adapted based on cause and stage of dementia, as well as the targeted goals, be they mood, agitation or memory recall. Connections to traumatic events can be inadvertently triggered in patients with memory loss, overstimulation can result from volume or instruments involved, or unknowing exposure to certain lyrics could worsen a depressed mood. Patients should be able to indicate their music preferences and their non-verbal responses to music should be monitored. These learnable skills could be reviewed periodically by a specialist in-home or via a tele-consultation.

Music therapy is too cost-effective an intervention not to be prioritised by most clinical and residential facilities managing dementia patients. Antipsychotics, the mainstay for dementia patient sedation, are statistically linked to increased risks for patient falls, stroke and even death. This, in turn, is associated with higher staff turnover and absence, although multiple factors likely play a role in this correlation. Music therapy cannot reverse the loss of cognitive function seen in dementia, but healthcare staff often perceive it as having positive direct and indirect impacts on their job satisfaction and express an interest in accessing more of such therapies for their patients. Increased access could result in overall improvements in job execution, even beyond direct care of their patients with dementia.

Text 1: Questions 7–14

7. In Paragraph 1, what does '**these**' refer to?

    (A) Mental abilities that are lost

    (B) Depression and anxiety

    (C) Drug preparations

    (D) Complementary therapies

8. In Paragraph 2, the author considers the ability of music to bypass normal processing centers of the brain to be

    (A) unexpected.

    (B) advantageous.

    (C) a hindrance.

    (D) not relevant.

9. The information in the Paragraph 3 suggests that

    (A) learning to play music is likely to become a cure for dementia.

    (B) selective chemical reactions in musicians' brains are protecting them.

    (C) any interaction with music can cause drastic changes in hormone levels.

    (D) persons can self-regulate their production of certain brain hormones.

10. The purpose of the information in the Paragraph 4 is to show

    (A) why comparing outcomes of diverse studies is difficult.

    (B) how outdated much of the research is.

    (C) which study designs offer the most reliable results.

    (D) that using professional therapists yields better outcomes.

11. What does the phrase, '**a faint light on the horizon**' imply?

- (A) There is still much to learn about how music affects the brain.
- (B) Optimised music therapies will still only provide small benefits for patients.
- (C) There is little hope of success because of practical obstacles.
- (D) Finding optimal therapy methods is possible, but much work is needed.

12. In Paragraph 5, the author makes the point that

- (A) family caregivers should have more options for home therapy.
- (B) caregiver well-being should receive more attention.
- (C) music therapy training for family caregivers should be more detailed.
- (D) music therapy support should be based on financial resources.

13. Paragraph 6 tells us that

- (A) incorrectly applied music therapy could accelerate cognitive decline.
- (B) a layman is unlikely to apply music therapy effectively.
- (C) music therapy is resource-friendly but requires technical skills.
- (D) permanent damage can result from incorrect music therapy.

14. In the final paragraph, what positive outcome does the author highlight?

- (A) Decrease in patient falls
- (B) Improved dementia outcomes
- (C) More efficient personnel functioning
- (D) Employment of more staff

Text 2: Pet Obesity

The prevalence of obesity in domestic pets has increased over the last 30 years, most notably in dogs and cats. An animal's level of body fat and overall nutrition status is assessed using the body condition score (BSC), with 1 indicating undernourishment and emaciation, and 9 indicating obesity. According to one 2017 US study by Banfield Pet Hospital, the number of dogs scoring 8 or higher on an obesity scale of 1–9 rose from 10% in 2007 to 19% in 2018, and the same category for cats rose from 19% to 34% over the same period. Equally concerning is that obesity was highest in juveniles, that is, 12–13 months old for cats and 24 months old for dogs, which are the key growth phases of these species.

Amongst dogs, those most impacted by obesity are small and so-called 'toy breeds' such as pugs, beagles and corgis. In cats, mixed-breed felines are at greatest risk, with genetics also being a risk factor for obesity. In many cases, these pets can extend even beyond the BSC scale, with animals at more than 40% above their ideal body weight. Yet owners often underestimate the true condition of their pet, possibly due to their perception of body shape being influenced by repeated exposure to other overweight pets, including even some in national show competitions. This **dissonance** can result in owners' distrust of professional assessment of their pet's nutritional status and attempts to intervene.

Beyond certain pure and mixed breeds being genetically predisposed to obesity, other factors play a role. Pets living indoors with less access to outdoor spaces are vulnerable to weight gain, highlighting the importance of a planned exercise regimen. Neutering changes sex-hormone balance, decreasing the desire for exertion while increasing food-seeking behaviours. The preplanned nature of neutering presents an opportunity to implement obesity-prevention strategies before the procedure. Co-existing diseases impact energy exchange and predisposal to weight gain. But by far the most consistent risk identified is too many treats, pre-packaged or family table scraps, something that can certainly be rationed.

Owners do play a role in their pets developing obesity, even in the face of animal risk factors. There is increased prevalence of pet obesity in households with lower-than-average income, overweight humans, humans spending less time actively interacting with pets and/or over-humanising of pets. Owner loneliness and depression, where the animal substitutes for human companionship, is an added challenge given that collaboration between animal and human doctors is not yet the norm. Yet it is pivotal that vets develop holistic, collaborative strategies as early as possible in the human-pet relationship and continue to promote these practices throughout the pet's life.

Many veterinarians resist conversations about obesity with owners because of the stigma associated with the condition. Alternatively, those keen to intervene may broach the subject without awareness of their own unconscious biases and of the impact their language may have on owners and outcomes. An example is the perception that owners who are obese are actually *causing* their pet's obesity, and that these owners will likely not comply with any recommendations anyway. This thinking goes against the fact that multiple risk factors contribute to pet obesity. Veterinarians should take an active and consistent approach to tackling all obesity and to the information that is available to them, so as to improve credibility, concordance and compliance.

Research has shown a negative correlation between body-fat mass and weight-loss success. Even with owner education and restricted calorie intake, animals typically lose less than 1% of their body fat per week across populations regardless of age, breed and neutering status. The inclusion of pets who are severely overweight and who often have a comorbidity such as arthritis, kidney disease or diabetes, contributes to **this**. Compliance with weight-loss strategies is usually good in the first 12 weeks, but few animals ever reach their ideal weight within this timeframe, and nearly 50% will subsequently regain weight. This emphasises the need for prevention and lifelong management.

A shift in thinking would likely prove more fruitful than the current focus on grammes lost. For prevention, growth-chart monitoring of juvenile body weight every 3–6 months could identify abnormal patterns early so that prevention strategies can be implemented. Online or telephone consultations with at-home weighing could be feasible substitutes when clinic visits are not. For already overweight pets, a focus on owner priorities may improve trust in advice and compliance. An owner may be more concerned about their dog's osteoarthritis and inability to run, and goals of improving mobility and decreasing pain would still incorporate weight loss. Grammes lost could be replaced by results gained in a set time (for example, in 12 weeks), at the end of which outcomes are reassessed and the owners' further priorities addressed.

Approaches to treating other chronic conditions such as osteoarthritis, diabetes and cardiopulmonary disease may also benefit from being **turned on their heads**. Traditionally, symptoms are treated first or tests are done that confirm a diagnosis and medicines given for that disease to achieve quick wins. But these strategies often mask the root cause of disease and only address any existing obesity as an afterthought. Yet losing excess body fat and increasing lean muscle improve most chronic diseases, and diet controls that relieve symptoms often state weight loss as a side effect. Meanwhile, short-term clinical gains from treating symptoms only can lead to long-term losses in terms of quality of life and longevity.

15. What is the author's main aim in Paragraph 1?

- (A) To educate about important maturation phases in cats and dogs.
- (B) To explain how animal fat and lean mass are calculated.
- (C) To suggest optimal timing for obesity interventions in certain animals.
- (D) To highlight the scale of the animal obesity problem.

16. In Paragraph 2, the '**dissonance**' mentioned refers to

- (A) how veterinarians judge animal status versus how owners judge it.
- (B) pure-breed dogs versus mixed-breed cats being the most affected.
- (C) how owners compare their pets to animals seen in contests.
- (D) interventions needed in severe obesity compared to those in moderate obesity.

17. What do we learn about pet obesity prevention in Paragraph 3?

- (A) Breed mixes that increase obesity risk should be avoided.
- (B) Many risk factors actually present opportunities for obesity prevention.
- (C) If done early enough, neutering will always prevent obesity.
- (D) Withholding treats and human food is the most recommended tactic.

18. What problem does the author outline in Paragraph 4?

- (A) Convincing owners to participate in obesity-management programmes.
- (B) Recognising contributing mental health issues in pet owners.
- (C) Collaborating with physicians for humans to effect outcomes.
- (D) Vet skills in developing comprehensive treatment plans.

19. In Paragraph 5, the author suggests that professionals should

- (A) adapt the advice they give based on pet-owner characteristics.
- (B) reassure owners that they are not responsible for their pet's obesity.
- (C) impress on pet owners that obesity should not be stigmatised.
- (D) examine their own prejudices before counselling owners of obese pets.

20. In Paragraph 6, '**this**' refers to

- (A) presence of a comorbidity.
- (B) weight-loss data.
- (C) programme compliance.
- (D) regaining weight.

21. In Paragraph 7, the author expresses

- (A) surprise that a focus on grammes lost has not been effective.
- (B) confidence that a change in thinking would improve owner interest.
- (C) disappointment that owners do not trust the advice of professionals.
- (D) frustration that telephone and online consultations are not exploited more.

22. In the final paragraph, the term '**turned on their heads**' refers to

- (A) doing full-spectrum testing for all chronic illnesses.
- (B) recommending weight loss in all chronically ill pets.
- (C) insisting owners take the lead in preventing obesity.
- (D) prioritising an approach that has traditionally been relegated.

End of Part C

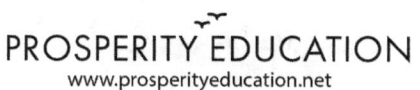

Occupational English Test

Reading

Test 6

Part A

- Look at the four texts (**A–D**) in the accompanying **text booklet**.
- For each question (**1–20**) look through the texts (**A–D**) to find the relevant information.
- Write your answers in the spaces provided in this **question paper**.
- Answer all the questions within the 15-minute time limit.
- Your answers should **only** be taken from texts **A–D** and must be correctly spelt.

Administration of Radiographic Contrast Medium: Questions

Questions 1–7

For each question (**1–7**), decide which text (**A, B, C** or **D**) the information comes from. Write the letter **A, B, C** or **D** in the space provided. You may use any letter more than once.

In which text can you find information about

1. drug options for preparing patients who may react negatively to contrast? _____

2. kinds of patients likely to have a negative reaction to contrast? _____

3. categorisation of adverse reactions? _____

4. a rare organ response in which the underlying cause is sometimes unclear? _____

5. types of catheters appropriate for contrast-medium infusions? _____

6. how to manage urgent patients at risk of adverse contrast reactions? _____

7. optimal technique to prevent damage to veins? _____

Questions 8–14

Answer each of the questions (**8–14**) with a word or short phrase from one of the texts. Each answer may include words, numbers or both. You should **not** write full sentences.

8. What should patients who are anxious receive before contrast is administered?

   _____

9. What drug can be given as premedication if IV methylprednisolone is contraindicated?

   _____

10 What serious disorder can occur in patients with either a compromised or normal heart?

_____

11 Pressure of the needle against the inside of the vein may prevent what?

_____

12 What size cannula is favoured for a contrast flow rate of 5ml every second?

_____

13 Which adult group has a much smaller chance of adverse reactions to contrast?

_____

14 How many doses of prednisone should be given in oral premedication?

_____

Questions 15–20

Complete each of the sentences (**15–20**) with a word or short phrase from one of the texts. Each answer may include words, numbers or both.

15 To decide how to proceed in non-severe reactions, _____ is needed.

16 Non-contrast allergies can pose as low as _____ risk of adverse reaction to contrast.

17 In moderate allergic reactions, shortness of breath does not accompany _____.

18 Contrast medium can still be given if the risk of adverse reaction is _____.

19 _____ can be omitted if premedication consists of methylprednisolone by mouth.

20 There is a danger of _____ when using thicker contrast fluids.

End of Part A

Administration of Radiographic Contrast Medium: Texts

Text A

Patient Screening

The highest predictive risk for adverse reactions to contrast medium is prior allergic-like reaction to the same class of medium. These patients have a roughly five-fold increased risk. There is, however, no cross-reactivity between different classes of contrast medium: a previous reaction to gadolinium-based contrast does not increase risk of future reaction to iodinated contrast, or vice versa. Children and the elderly have much lower reaction rates than middle-aged persons, and males much lower than females.

Non-contrast-related allergies* have a zero- to three-fold higher risk of adverse reactions when compared to the general population. For example, shellfish allergies pose no greater risk.

Medical conditions associated with some increased risk:

- Asthma*
- Renal insufficiency – patient screening is aimed at mitigating nephrotoxicity or systemic fibrosis, which can be triggered by contrasts, as opposed to an allergic reaction.
- Cardiac disease (e.g. severe aortic stenosis, cardiac arrhythmias) – if an adverse reaction does occur, there is an increased chance of a consequent cardiac event. Close monitoring is indicated.
- Myasthenia gravis* – may be considered a relative contraindication for contrast medium.
- Hyperthyroidism* – patients can develop thyrotoxicosis if given iodinated contrast medium, but this non-allergic complication is rare.

Other considerations

- Beta-blockers* may lower the threshold for contrast adverse reactions, increase reaction severity, and decrease responsiveness to epinephrine given for allergic reactions, but evidence is inconsistent. Beta-blocker therapy can continue prior to contrast medium administration.
- Anxiety – there is some evidence that contrast reactions are more common in anxious patients. Reassurance before injections may lessen chances of mild contrast reactions.

*Indicated conditions have modest increased risk. However, restricting contrast use or premedicating solely on these bases is not recommended.

Text B

Premedication

Premedication aims to mitigate the likelihood of an allergic-like reaction in high-risk patients. It does not prevent all reactions, and use in high-risk patients should be assessed individually. Regimens of 2 hours or less (oral or IV; corticosteroid- or antihistamine-based) are largely ineffective.

Administration Route	Duration	Indications	Regimen
Oral	12–13 hours	Outpatient with a prior adverse reaction to the same class of contrast medium (e.g. iodinated –> iodinated).	50mg prednisone at 13 hours, 7 hours, and 1 hour before contrast administration + 50mg diphenhydramine 1 hour before contrast administration OR 2mg methylprednisolone 12 hours and 2 hours before contrast given (optional: 50mg diphenhydramine may be added)
		Emergency Room patient or inpatient with a prior adverse reaction to the same contrast class (e.g. iodinated –> iodinated) and in whom premedication will not negatively delay care.	
Intravenous	4–5 hour 'accelerated regimen' found to be efficacious	Outpatient with a prior adverse reaction to the same contrast class, who has not been premedicated and cannot be easily rebooked.	Commence with methylprednisolone 40mg or hydrocortisone 200mg, then every 4 hours until contrast given + diphenhydramine 50mg 1 hour before contrast given. OR (If methylprednisolone allergy) Immediately, dexamethasone 7.5mg, then every 4 hours until contrast given + diphenhydramine 50mg 1 hour before contrast given.
		Emergency department patient or inpatient with a prior reaction to the same contrast class, in whom 12- or 13-hour premedication will negatively delay care.	
		Patients unable to take oral medication	

Text C

Contrast Medium Administration By Power Injector

It should not be assumed that the power injector can be used with all central-venous catheter tubing. Catheter manufacturers' guidelines should be adhered to. Power injectors should not be used with small-bore access (e.g. for access points at the wrist or hand). Venipuncture sites require the use of a flexible plastic cannula; metal needles should be avoided whenever possible. Contrast flow rate depends on needle gauge. 20G or larger cannula is preferred for flow rates over 3ml/sec. However, the smaller 22G may tolerate flow rates up to 5ml/sec.

Technique

An antecubital or large forearm vein is preferred. If a more peripheral venipuncture site is used, flow rates should be reduced.

1. Clear the power injector contrast syringe and pressure tubing of air. The tubing attached to the contrast syringe should be kept orientated downward.

2. Insert venous cannula at a properly prepared venipuncture site (ideally, large vein of the forearm).

3. After insertion, check cannula positioning for backflow of blood, which indicates correct positioning. Backflow may be blocked if the cannula tip is pressed against the internal wall of the vein.

4. Vein flushing with saline can be performed manually with a standard syringe or using the power injector saline function.

5. If the venipuncture site is found to be tender or infiltrated during flushing, an alternative site should be sought.

The use of viscous contrast medium increases risk of extravasation. Minimise risk by using flexible plastic cannulas instead of metal needles, employing a meticulous venous cannula insertion technique and securing the cannula to the patient's skin.

Text D

Acute Adverse Reactions

ACUTE ADVERSE REACTIONS

Assessment of reaction severity is subjective. Clinical judgment is needed to determine how aggressively to intervene in mild and moderate cases.

- Mild: self-treatment or resolves during clinical observation.
- Moderate: usually require medical attention. May progress to severe.
- Severe: can be life-threatening or cause permanent morbidity. Pulmonary edema is a rare severe reaction that can occur in patients with fragile cardiac reserve or normal cardiac function. If the etiology is unclear, assume that the reaction is allergic in nature.

ALLERGIC (immune system-mediated)

Mild	Moderate	Severe
• Discrete urticaria	• Diffuse urticaria & pruritis	• Facial oedema with dyspnoea
• Skin oedema	• Diffuse erythema; pulse, BP and respiration stable	• Generalised erythema with hypotension
• 'scratchy' throat	• Facial swelling without dyspnoea	• Laryngeal oedema with stridor
• Sneezing, conjunctivitis, rhinorrhea	• Throat tightness	• Bronchospasm + hypoxia
	• Wheezing	• Hypotension + tachycardia
	• Mild or absent hypoxia	

PHYSIOLOGIC (direct effect on organs)

Mild	Moderate	Severe
• Limited nausea or vomiting	• Protracted nausea & vomiting	• Fainting, not readily responsive to treatment
• Transient flushing / warmth / chills	• Hypertension	• Arrhythmias
• Headache, dizziness / nervousness	• Isolated chest pain	• Seizures
• Mild hypertension	• Fainting responsive to treatment	• Hypertensive crisis
• Transient fainting resolving spontaneously		

End of Part A | Text booklet

Part B

In this part of the test, there are six short extracts relating to the work of health professionals. For questions **1–6**, choose the answer (**A, B or C**) that you think fits best according to the text.

Your answers should be made by filling in the circle completely: Ⓐ

1. What does the manual say about bed-cleaning agents?

    Ⓐ They should only be used in concentrations of 10% or less.

    Ⓑ Cleaning mattresses requires longer drying times than cleaning bed frames.

    Ⓒ Not all bed cleaning should make use of regular household products.

MANUAL: CLEANING OF PATIENT ADVANCED BEDS
Bed Frame
To access under the bed frame for cleaning, manually lift the foot end of the frame until the latch mechanism securely engages, or, similarly, lift the head end of the frame.
Mattress
To minimise exposure to harsh chemicals, general cleaning of the sleep-surface mattress cover can include wiping with a sponge or rag dampened in a standard household quaternary ammonium-type cleaner. Cleaning solutions should be used and diluted according to the manufacturer's instructions.
The Clorox Broad Spectrum® brand of industrial-strength cleaner should be reserved for situations where deep disinfection is needed, and should be used in concentrations no greater than 1 part in 10 parts of water. Special care should be taken to remove all excess disinfecting solution. Allow a minimum of 30 minutes in a well-ventilated space for cleaned areas to dry.

2. According to the guidelines

   (A) a deteriorated sample should be properly discarded as soon as possible.

   (B) a sample that has deteriorated during transport may still be tested.

   (C) rejected samples should be stored for review of the reasons for rejection.

Laboratory Sample Rejection

Samples for testing should be properly labelled, adequate in quantity and appropriate for the test requested. Rejection of samples can be due to:
- missing or illegible labels
- insufficient patient information
- damaged containers or covers
- insufficient specimen
- poor storage during transport or hemolysis in tests requiring intact red cells
- collection in the wrong colour-coded container

If a sample is rejected, the doctor submitting the sample should be contacted immediately and another sample requested. The original sample should be retained pending decision about its disposal, proceeding with testing despite the sample not being optimal, or receipt of a new specimen.

Management should regularly review reasons for sample rejection, conduct appropriate training and revise written procedures for sample collection and handling.

3. What do the medico-legal guidelines make clear about deaths in presumed criminal poisoning?

(A) The medical team can discard any patient items they believe are not related to the death.

(B) The doctor is not obligated to tell the family the reason for withholding the death certificate.

(C) In all cases of poisoning, only a physician can directly report the information to the police.

Physicians' Duty In Suspected Criminal Poisoning
When attending a patient suspected of having been intentionally poisoned, physicians have a duty of patient care but must also make accurate, detailed notes, collect potential evidence and take responsibility for ensuring that the local police are promptly informed. If patient fatality has occurred, the physician must withhold completion of the death certificate, relay to the next of kin only that it is being withheld and the police should be informed of the death.
The physician's report should include details of: • patient demographic data • date and time of presentation and/or death • description of all organ systems • treatment given and patient response.
Any biological materials should be preserved, including stomach contents as well as any circumstantial evidence such as clothing or items suspected of having had contact with the poison.

4. The Recertification Guidelines inform dietitians that they

   (A) cannot rollover or redo incomplete recertification activities in another cycle.

   (B) are audited in the order in which their documentation was received.

   (C) cannot access recertification activities before confirming certain professional criteria.

Recertification Guidelines For Dietitians

Qualified dietitians are required to update their Professional Development Portfolio (PDP) once per 5-year cycle in order to maintain their certification.

When recertifying, practitioners must first submit documentation attesting to meeting clinical practice requirements. They will then be able to update their PDP for updating and submission.

Recertification activities for updating are listed in your account. Activities started but not completed in the last 6 months of a recertification cycle may be credited to the next cycle. All activities started prior to this window must be completed within that cycle or restarted in the next cycle.

Updated portfolios are audited randomly. Dietitians are advised to retain audit documentation for a minimum of 2 years beyond the end of the recertification period.

5. What does the protocol say about handling used linen?

(A) There are multiple acceptable ways to sanitise linen.

(B) It should be washed immediately.

(C) By law, it should never be placed on the floor.

Handling Hospital Used Linen
It is a legislative requirement that staff handling used linen wear personal protective equipment (PPE), such as disposable plastic aprons and gloves, and hand hygiene must be performed after handling used linen. Handling recommendations for used items aim to minimise cross contamination: do not hold used linen against your person or place used linen on the floor, and materials should be agitated as little as possible.
Linen being stored until a viable complete load has been gathered for transportation or cleaning should be in color-coded hampers in a designated storage area that is inaccessible to the public and locked when not attended by staff.
Laundering should include a disinfection cycle using a cleaning agent and water above 60° Celsius. Over 65° Celsius, minimum disinfection cycle lengths vary from 3–25 minutes, as shown in the attached table. Cold cycles require the addition of a bleach agent, but this may not kill all microorganisms.

6. Recommendations in the text include

    (A) initial discussion about how the patient can become independent in their therapy.

    (B) setting limits on physiotherapy consultations during the first visit.

    (C) outlining how carers can be trained to take the role of the physiotherapist.

Physiotherapy In Parkinson's Disease

Formal physiotherapy appointments do not need to be ongoing in Parkinson's. Self-managed therapy enables direct assessment of impact on activities of daily life, and carers can contribute in a more real-life context.

Physiotherapists should discuss and agree with patients as early as during history-taking how therapy will be continued after completion of the professional treatment period. Patients must consent to involvement of carers in sessions and can stipulate to what extent the carer is to be involved in self-managed therapy.

Periodic follow-up or monitoring appointments that are to occur during the self-managed phase should be covered. If a telephone number or email address is provided, agree who will originate the contact and its timing. The advice of allied health professionals (e.g. a dietitian or an occupational therapist) should also be incorporated, as appropriate.

End of Part B

Part C

In this part of the test, there are two texts about different aspects of healthcare. For questions **7–22**, choose the answer (**A, B, C** or **D**) that you think fits best according to the text.

Your answers should be made by filling in the circle completely: Ⓐ Ⓑ Ⓒ Ⓓ

Text 1: The Face Of Modern Malnutrition

In modern times, vitamin deficiency is often thought of as a problem of lower- and middle-income countries (LMICs), but increasingly it is being recognised as a current and persistent issue even in higher-income countries (HICs). Prior to the early 20th Century, goiters, anemia, rickets and pellagra were common micronutrient deficiencies seen by healthcare workers. Coordinated public health measures all but eliminated them from the public consciousness in affluent countries. However, modern food security in higher-income countries is being challenged by convenient energy-dense-but-vitamin-poor meals, lifestyles that sometimes limit sun exposure, and chronic diseases and treatment interventions that can hinder gut-micronutrient absorption. One study revealed a more than ten-fold rise in vitamin deficiencies among Europeans in the time frame from 2005 to 2015. And one in three Americans is said to have either a vitamin deficiency or anemia.

Regardless of setting, vitamin-deficiency burden tends to be highest in pregnant women, young children, adolescents and the elderly. LMIC pregnant women are especially vulnerable as poorer maternal diets result in low gestational weight gain, low birth weights, and failure to thrive and developmental issues in newborns. Additionally, inadequate obstetric care, close spacing of pregnancies and low education are risk factors in these settings where nutritional deficiencies are often overt and severe. In contrast, vitamin deficiencies in HICs are often covert, causing generic fatigue, frequent infections, impaired cognitive function and labile mood. Late intervention has implications for long-term health, with research showing links between vitamin deficiency and cardiovascular disease, diabetes mellitus, malignancies, osteoporosis and even age-related eye diseases.

Christina B, 47, lives in northern Germany. She first noticed sore gums and a maculo-papular rash on both wrists in 2019, which were attributed to stress caused by quitting smoking after 20 years. In the two years that followed, Christina experienced further skin changes, joint pains and poor wound healing after foot surgery. Finally, scurvy was diagnosed empirically and vitamin C-rich foods and supplements saw a turnaround in her condition. Similarly, in the tropical Caribbean, 56-year-old non-vegan Magareta S attended a locum GP for a refill of her hypertension medication, and mentioned persisting symptoms, namely thinning hair, altered sense of taste and increased fatigue, assessed by her regular GP as due to menopause. Blood tests instead confirmed B12 deficiency, and appropriate treatment was successfully implemented. Physicians in all settings must be alert to the possibility of vitamin deficiencies so that unnecessary suffering, cost and complications are avoided.

Vitamin C deficiency stands as an example of a micronutrient deficiency made ubiquitous by modern lifestyles. At high risk for scurvy are those who over-consume alcohol, have gastrointestinal disorders, such as inflammatory bowel disease, or are post-bariatric surgery, as well as smokers who have high free-radical levels that can overwhelm the oxidative capacity of available vitamin C, reduce its absorption in the gut and increase its excretion by the kidneys.

Those consuming higher levels of convenient junk food and lower quantities of fresh fruits and vegetables, or who have extreme diet restrictions are also vulnerable.

The World Health Organization estimates that 25% of the world's population has vitamin D deficiency. It is prevalent among Japanese women who traditionally avoid ultraviolet radiation on their skin and have a diet low in vitamin D. It is also seen among US adolescents who have hypertension, hyperglycemia and metabolic syndrome with or without adiposity. The ODIN project funded by the European Union is investigating the efficacy of improving vitamin D levels through food-fortification. Such a policy was introduced in Finland in 2003, targeting milk products specifcially, and recent data gathered by Tuija et al. confirms the success of the initiative. Other countries with comparable needs continue to fiercely debate the adoption of similar proven policies.

The B group of vitamins are essential for food metabolism, blood cell creation and preventing DNA damage, and checking that blood levels are adequate helps minimise risk of disease. B1 (thiamin) insufficiency is common in strict gluten-free and vegan diets, and nicotine consumption in the form of cigarettes, vaping or patches, and is worsened by alcohol abuse. Indeed, the role of average alcohol consumption in thiamin deficiency is underappreciated. Ethanol in alcohol blocks thiamin conversion to its active form, reducing its bioavailability by as much as 54%, while tannic acids in coffee, tea and energy drinks also impair absorption. And although polypharmacy is common, especially in the elderly, familiar drugs such as metformin and metronidazole inhibit thiamin uptake. Older people are also particularly susceptible to B12 malabsorption because of age-related gastrointestinal disorders.

It is said that 'most people can get all the vitamins they need from a healthy diet'. Yet maintaining a healthy diet is the challenge. Market forces have somehow come into play in what constitutes 'good health behaviours', with diets trending then fading, making micronutrient fortification more a **commercial dice game** than a scientific undertaking. Moreover, nutrition research is not lucrative, and it receives, on average, less than 5% of research budgets. Drug effects can be isolated by giving some study participants a placebo, but there are no placebos in diet research as bodies process nutrients differently and observing the effects of micronutrient balance takes decades. Public interest currently has veered to microbiomes and probiotics, and medications such as the weight-loss drug Ozempic produce fast, visual results that overshadow information about long-term effects of micronutrients.

Ironically, diet fortification and vitamin supplements carry at least a theoretical possibility of excess intake and toxicity. Any delay in diagnosis of micronutrient abnormalities increases chances of patient morbidity and psychological stress. Professional dietetic assessments can offer guidance on nutritional status with selective and appropriate treatment of micronutrient abnormalities. More cases of vitamin deficiencies in high-income countries have begun to surface in medical journals. **These** emphasise the importance of increased awareness and the need for specific screening protocols when encountering ambiguous clinical signs alongside suggestive clinical histories.

Text 1: Questions 7–14

7. In Paragraph 1, what does the author suggest about modern diets in HICs?

    A. Past experience with vitamin deficiencies has not addressed modern issues.

    B. Ample food supply has worsened the quality of modern western diets.

    C. Micronutrient deficits in affluent countries now equal those in LMICs.

    D. European and American diets produce the highest rates of vitamin deficiency.

8. What problem does the author identify in Paragraph 2?

    A. Teaching pregnant women about vitamin deficiencies is more challenging in LMICs.

    B. Not recognising low-grade vitamin deficiency can result in severe pathology.

    C. Non-dietary risk factors are responsible for the greater burden of illness.

    D. In HICs, patients are late in seeking help for diet-related illnesses.

9. In Paragraph 3, the author gives the patient examples mainly to emphasise

    A. the range of symptoms that can be caused by vitamin deficiency.

    B. the diverse geographical and ethnic profiles of vitamin deficiency.

    C. guidelines on investigating suspected nutrient deficiencies.

    D. that effective treatment often depends on an index of suspicion.

10. In Paragraph 4, vitamin C is used to exemplify

    A. one common cause of gut problems.

    B. a complex biological interaction between substances.

    C. why certain drugs should be avoided.

    D. an illness caused by routine personal behaviors.

11. The information in Paragraph 5 demonstrates that

    (A) effective interventions do not equal problem-solving unless adopted routinely.

    (B) it is hard to find a practicable vitamin D solution at national levels.

    (C) metabolic disorders are disproportionately high in US teens.

    (D) burdens of vitamin D deficiency are similar across all countries.

12. What do we learn about B vitamins in Paragraph 6?

    (A) Their deficiency is a major contributor to many chronic diseases.

    (B) Eating some vegetables can worsen certain vitamin B deficiencies.

    (C) Concurrent smoking and alcohol intake have a cumulative effect on bioavailability.

    (D) Prescribing multiple drugs may nullify the risk of vitamin B deficiencies.

13. The author uses the term '**commercial dice game**' to suggest that

    (A) profits and popular sentiment illogically drive ideas of good diet.

    (B) stakeholders are not serious about what nutrition research they support.

    (C) choosing to pursue nutrition research is financially high-risk.

    (D) it is very challenging to make big profits from nutrition initiatives.

14. '**These**' in the final paragraph refers to

    (A) nutritional evaluations.

    (B) micronutrient abnormalities.

    (C) case studies.

    (D) patient complications.

Text 2: The Ongoing Debate About Shift Length

Shift work can have individual consequences, including physiological, mental and social effects. The macroscopic view of healthcare systems, however, focuses on absenteeism rates, patient and staff safety, staff retention and overall institutional and health-sector costs. Individual impacts do receive much warranted attention, but it is the costs that ultimately determine the governing model of how healthcare personnel continue to work, including shiftwork. Currently, there is a lack of information on the specific impacts of shift work within homogeneous groups across a range of healthcare professions (HCP). This is needed to replace the existing mixed-research approaches, inconsistent study results and challenging interpretations, as cost considerations will remain intrinsically shaped by individual factors.

Atypical working hours have been shown to positively correlate with cardiovascular, metabolic and other disorders. Night work has been identified as one of the main causes of increased likelihood of workplace accidents due to fatigue, attention, memory and response-inhibition issues, with demonstrable deterioration over consecutive night shifts. However, some studies suggest that **these** can be mitigated by adapting the circadian rhythm of shift workers. Work by Leso et al. in 2021 and also by both Chang and Kazemi suggest that subjects working seven consecutive night shifts adapt better than those working four consecutive night shifts. Meanwhile, more recent studies propose rotating every two or three days to reduce the frequency of the body's need to adjust.

Healthcare personnel have historically been less likely than other professionals to acknowledge that shift work and fatigue might affect their performance, with nurses and doctors often viewing themselves as 'super-human': able to work optimally for long hours without breaks, food or hydration. This mindset itself **skates on thin ice**. The COVID-19 pandemic laid bare the urgent need for monitoring personnel fatigue and the value of taking action before safety risk and burnout occur. This approach has direct implications for staff as well as institutional health. Risk-assessment tools already exist in other sectors such as aviation. Their tools cannot be directly adopted by the healthcare industry because of its differing job demands, but they could help to inform development and deployment of similar tools in the health workplace.

Nurses working shifts of 12–13 hours are reported to be more likely to experience burnout and leave the profession than those working 8–9-hour shifts. Yet many nurses have more subjectively favourable views towards longer shifts because of the lower number of consecutive shifts and potentially better work-life balance. Administrative arguments in favour of longer shifts include improved continuity of patient care due to fewer handovers and lower institution costs from less shift overlap. Conversely, longer shifts with more consecutive days off have been linked to staff working beyond the end of a shift, decreased opportunities for educational development activities and feeling less connected to colleagues, the latter point raised especially among night shift and part-time HCP. Facts gleaned from larger personnel samples, more assessment parameters and comparable study designs are currently needed to better inform policy.

In terms of patient care, results are inconsistent. Some suggest that patient safety may deteriorate with a 12-hour shift system, and there is no irrefutable proof that continuity of patient care really is improved with longer shifts. But there is consistency with respect to patient satisfaction. In 2012, Stimpel et al. found that as the proportion of hospital nurses working shifts of 13 hours or more increased, so did patients' dissatisfaction with their care. This has borne out still in 2024, in a meta-analysis by Zixin Li et al. scoping 85 studies across 32 countries and nearly 300,000 nurses. Yet Zixin Li still found that instances of patient complaints, patient abuse and mortality rates did not increase regardless of other factors such as nurse age, work experience or geography, findings that could be seized upon by HCP to justify viewing themselves as 'super-human', and by financial decision-makers who wish to only consider the universal perspective.

Worldwide, there is a shortage of nearly 6 million nurses and 4 million doctors in locations in need, with a struggle to entice younger generations into the sector. Increased on-the-job demands and burnout have skyrocketed staff-turnover rates. Financial gains from longer shifts may already be decimated by costs associated with personnel burnout, sick leave, resignations and recruitment. Currently, recruiting a registered nurse can cost over $50,000, and a doctor over $100,000. Given the time needed to fully train a nurse or doctor, there is little wonder that increasing numbers of temporary staff and assistants are being introduced into the deficit. Cost-effectiveness, therefore, must focus more broadly on where and how expenditure for shifts is allocated. And if 12-hour shifts are to remain, individual risks such as reduced productivity and efficiency, burnout and resignations must be incorporated into policies around schedules and support.

Giving nurses increased control over shift patterns has been explored as a way to reduce sickness absence, and has been found to be effective when compared to traditional scheduling systems. Nurse managers could further foster a culture that does not discourage staff reporting fatigue so that precautions can be implemented to avoid workplace accidents and burnout. Prompt departure at the end of a shift should be encouraged wherever possible, and days off and vacation time requests respected. At top levels of the hierarchy, legislation could require organisations to show that workers are aware of scheduling policies and understand the implications of longer shifts. Furthermore, standardised monitoring and recording of absenteeism, accidents and reports of increased fatigue could be implemented so that effects at the employee, patient-care and finance levels could be better collated across institutions.

15. What aspect of data on shift work is highlighted in Paragraph 1?

- (A) The low level of attention financial planners give to employee perspectives.
- (B) The need to gather more data from personnel when optimising costs.
- (C) The largely negative nature of the impact of shiftwork on staff.
- (D) The wide range of studies available from which reliable data can be gathered.

16. In Paragraph 2, the word '**these**' refers to

- (A) studies on impacts of shift work.
- (B) the findings of Leso, Chang and Kazemi.
- (C) atypical and night-working hours.
- (D) physiological and cognitive disruptions.

17. In Paragraph 2, what does the author suggest about studies on optimal shift-change rates?

- (A) They are contradictory, with earlier studies promoting a slower shift change rate.
- (B) A gradual decrease in shift length from seven to two days helps adaptation.
- (C) A 24-hour off-duty period between shift changes is the optimal rest time.
- (D) Those working seven-day shift rotations experience less fatigue.

18. The phrase '**skates on thin ice**' refers to

- (A) the increase chance of health professionals collapsing from fatigue.
- (B) professionals being less aware of the danger they can pose.
- (C) personnel being accustomed to working optimally for longer periods.
- (D) professionals being resistant to the idea of being monitored.

19. The author's main goal in Paragraph 4 is to

- (A) highlight the optimal shift length to minimise negative effects on workers.
- (B) demonstrate why the assumptions of healthcare managers are likely wrong.
- (C) show that assessment of shift impact must focus on multiple factors.
- (D) list the limited number of issues shift workers really care about.

20. In Paragraph 5, the author expresses

- (A) wariness that Li's results may be used to keep detrimental shift patterns.
- (B) shock that patient-complaint and death rates are not higher with longer shifts.
- (C) disappointment at the weak existing evidence around patient safety and satisfaction.
- (D) skepticism that results in 2024 remain so similar to those from 2012.

21. In Paragraph 6, the author makes the point that

- (A) too much is being spent on the recruitment of qualified professionals.
- (B) there is an increased cost to using temporary staff and assistants.
- (C) there should be more drives to recruit youngsters into health professions.
- (D) overall profits from longer shifts may be much less than assumed.

22. What is the author doing in the final paragraph?

- (A) Highlighting initiatives that have decreased sick days at other institutions
- (B) Pointing out areas in which nurse managers have traditionally fallen short
- (C) Suggesting practicable measures to empower and support nurses
- (D) Describing a data-collection tool that would yield more reliable statistics

End of Part C

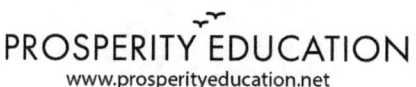

Answers

Test 1 | Answer key

Part A

#	Ans		#	Ans	
1	C		11	C	vomiting
2	C		12	A	timely follow up
3	D		13	D	cognitive behavioural counseling
4	B		14	D	two / 2 weeks
5	A		15	C	miscarriage
6	C		16	D	pleasure
7	D		17	A	evidence-based / evidence based
8	D	varenicline	18	B	one to three / 1-to-3 / 1–3 days
9	C	one to two / 1-to-2 / 1–2 hours	19	C	bradycardia
10	B	ten / 10 seconds	20	D	sensitive

Part B

#	Ans		#	Ans	
1	B	two staff members are needed to manoeuvre a patient if using a ceiling-lift device.	4	C	the programme will reduce the risks to patients.
2	A	the admitting physician is not automatically qualified to verify patient EIP self-management.	5	C	give guidelines on the correct maintenance schedule for the station.
3	B	identify which drugs can go into household waste and which need special considerations.	6	A	persons not related to the dementia patient can play a role in determining if the dementia patient can give their own consent.

Part C

#	Ans		#	Ans	
7	D	show how research in this area has evolved over time	15	B	is ambivalent about whether NPs do achieve better health outcomes
8	C	starting to tackle grief even before the dying person has passed away	16	B	a large number of patients can benefit from naturopathy
9	A	they associate grief with self-perceived failure to extend life	17	A	an example of ineffective ingredients in accepted medicines
10	C	doctors were not obligated to attend grief-training programmes	18	D	help readers make informed decisions about alternative therapies
11	A	unintentionally highlights why physician grief can become complicated	19	C	reiterate the ongoing problems with getting data on alternative therapies
12	D	the classic stages of grief	20	A	displace the current stakeholders and value system
13	D	a lack of substantial prospective study data	21	B	the general public has broader definitions for what it accepts as proof
14	B	it has taken too long for the emotional limitations of doctors to be acknowledged	22	C	misuse the naturopathy title

Test 2 | Answer key

Part A					
1	B		11	D	drug treatment options OR drug options
2	C		12	A	1-2% OR one to two percent
3	A		13	B	neovascularization OR neovascularisation
4	A		14	C	patch (the) eyes
5	D		15	B	Pseudomonas OR pseudomonas
6	B		16	C	41 weeks
7	D		17	D	from nose to ear
8	C	25mg/kg / OR 25mg per kg	18	A	cervix and urethra
9	C	(the) same day	19	C	pyloric stenosis
10	B	throat, rectum OR throat & rectum	20	B	slightly bloody

Part B					
1	B	may be used for teaching students	4	A	staff must remove their uniforms before smoking regular or e-cigarettes
2	A	the physician must first see the patient face-to-face	5	C	help clinical facilities to update their patient-management approach
3	C	must be used at some point when communicating with the patient	6	C	the Emergency Department used to experience the most lawsuits

Part C					
7	A	show why the disease might be unreported	15	D	the lack of studies on team multiculturalism
8	B	both positive and negative aspects of tackling the infection	16	B	there is some merit to giving patients the kind of staff member they want
9	A	multiple tiers in society are responsible for dengue spread	17	A	demonstrate the wide personal and professional impacts of good teamwork
10	D	demonstrate specific situations where education is needed	18	C	how individual experience can impact the wider sector
11	D	the distribution of the 2023 outbreak in Peru	19	B	provide a good template for a healthcare model
12	C	decreasing the numbers of mosquitoes in some ways did more harm than good	20	A	the power structure might inhibit the goals they want to achieve
13	B	protecting even a small percentage of persons from dengue is a significant achievement	21	D	allows for development of intercultural skills
14	A	worries that the virus may find new ways to spread	22	A	hiring decisions should be guided by commercial revenue data

Test 3 | Answer key

Part A

#	Ans		#	Ans	
1	C		11	C	bedaquiline
2	D		12	B	(approximately) 37%
3	A		13	C	2000mg / 2g
4	A		14	A	eighteen / 18 times
5	B		15	A	brassy
6	C		16	B	reassurance
7	B		17	D	cachexia
8	B	Mantoux (technique)	18	C	shortest protocol
9	A	growth points	19	C	pre-mixed formulations
10	D	set an alert	20	D	drug resistance

Part B

#	Ans		#	Ans	
1	B	that not all drug interactions must be avoided.	4	C	to consider multiple factors when assessing patient motivation for gift-giving.
2	C	parents/guardians can stop or change the resuscitation efforts during the process.	5	B	patients may be denied home oxygen therapy even if it is strongly indicated clinically.
3	A	to outline the procedure for handling patient belongings.	6	A	saying you are sorry after an accident can negatively affect your claim.

Part C

#	Ans		#	Ans	
7	D	general knowledge and demands for more help for autism	15	C	the One Health ideology utilises a strategic approach
8	A	rethinking definitions of autism has made it a more common diagnosis	16	B	individuals supporting changes needed
9	D	demonstrates why available data should not be taken at face value	17	B	neglecting to invest in preventive public health measures
10	B	the ability to compensate for one behaviour by using another	18	D	to outline the monumental scope of the One Health undertaking
11	C	found similar results to other studies done before	19	B	current and future health challenges are a result of human scientific advancement
12	A	acknowledges that there are drawbacks to ABA therapy	20	A	misses a crucial element needed to make it viable
13	A	neurodiversity supporters	21	C	convinced communities will need externally imposed objective guidelines and definitions.
14	C	the two sides agree on some aspects of the autism debate	22	B	poorer countries will remain behind despite One Health's goals

Test 4 | Answer key

Part A

#	Ans		#	Ans	
1	D		11	B	deferoxamine
2	C		12	A	38C/Centigrade/Celsius and above
3	A		13	B	mid-stream / midstream / MSU
4	D		14	C	intranasal diamorphine
5	B		15	A	antiemetics and laxatives
6	B		16	B	unhelpful
7	C		17	D	cell turnover
8	B	HbS	18	A	main care physician
9	A	(a/the) triage nurse	19	B	1% / one percent / 1 percent
10	D	bedwetting	20	C	10 kg / ten kilograms

Part B

#	Ans		#	Ans	
1	C	Only certain ulcers should be detailed on the pressure ulcer form.	4	A	A list of the fixed-weight additional bed items should be kept.
2	C	Administration of palliative care should continue.	5	B	are not permitted to access social media during work hours when in the hospital.
3	A	outline the main areas to be checked during a heatwave.	6	C	Clinicians can document domestic abuse even when it is not confirmed.

Part C

#	Ans		#	Ans	
7	B	pragmatic about the range of concerns being raised.	15	C	errors in the data Quetelet used.
8	D	corrective material that has been attached to the vector.	16	D	shows definite validity for a specific parameter.
9	B	The hazards of GT are less persuasive than their benefits.	17	C	emphasise shortcomings in the calculation of BMI.
10	C	what the media highlights.	18	D	BMI documentation might be out of habit rather than need.
11	A	how a highly effective drug can fail to help patients.	19	A	why BMI alone should not be the basis for treatment
12	B	The way the trials were designed.	20	B	facing potential difficulties after receiving unqualified health assessments.
13	C	use public domain processes.	21	B	It is a more robust health indicator than BMI.
14	A	People may receive GT made specifically for them.	22	A	healthcare should seek help from outside the sector

Test 5 | Answer key

Part A

#	Ans		#	Ans	
1	C		11	B	4 / four months
2	D		12	A	keratinised plugs
3	C		13	D	liver and spleen
4	A		14	C	intralesional
5	A		15	B	antacids
6	B		16	A	virilising
7	B		17	C	urgent
8	D	topical (acne) (treatment/treatments)	18	D	fluctuating
9	C	sinus tracts	19	C	fillers
10	A	1% / one percent / 1 percent	20	B	spironolactone

Part B

#	Ans		#	Ans	
1	A	does not have to pre-approve all out-of-network referrals.	4	C	the rules governing how and when strikes occur.
2	A	a particular directional hair-removal technique.	5	C	can advise an affected patient to continue taking the recalled drug.
3	B	Medically prescribed bed rest prior to testing could invalidate glucose results.	6	B	had similar diagnoses and higher than recommended drug doses.

Part C

#	Ans		#	Ans	
7	C	Drug preparations	15	D	To highlight the scale of the animal obesity problem.
8	B	Advantageous.	16	A	how veterinarians judge animal status versus how owners judge it.
9	B	selective chemical reactions in musicians' brains are protecting them	17	B	Many risk factors actually present opportunities for obesity prevention.
10	A	why comparing outcomes of diverse studies is difficult.	18	C	Collaborating with physicians for humans to effect outcomes.
11	D	Finding optimal therapy methods is possible, but much work is needed.	19	D	examine their own prejudices before counselling owners of obese pets.
12	B	caregiver well-being should receive more attention.	20	B	weight-loss data.
13	C	music therapy is resource-friendly but requires technical skills.	21	B	confidence that a change in thinking would improve owner interest.
14	C	More efficient personnel functioning	22	D	prioritising an approach that has traditionally been relegated.

Test 6 | Answer key

Part A

#	Ans		#	Ans	
1	B		11	C	backflow / back-flow / back flow
2	A		12	C	20G or larger / 20 gauge or larger
3	D		13	A	(the) (male) elderly
4	D		14	B	3 / three
5	C		15	D	clinical judgement
6	B		16	A	zero / 0
7	C		17	D	facial swelling
8	A	reassurance	18	A	modest
9	B	dexamethasone	19	B	(50mg) diphenhydramine
10	D	pulmonary edema / oedema	20	C	extravasation

Part B

#	Ans		#	Ans	
1	C	Not all bed cleaning should make use of regular household products.	4	C	cannot access recertification activities before confirming certain professional criteria.
2	B	a sample that has deteriorated during transport may still be tested.	5	A	There are multiple acceptable ways to sanitise linen.
3	B	The doctor is not obligated to tell the family the reason for withholding the death certificate.	6	A	initial discussion about how the patient can become independent in their therapy.

Part C

#	Ans		#	Ans	
7	A	Past experience with vitamin deficiencies has not addressed modern issues.	15	B	The need to gather more data from personnel when optimising costs.
8	B	Not recognising low-grade vitamin deficiency can result in severe pathology.	16	D	physiological and cognitive disruptions.
9	D	that effective treatment often depends on an index of suspicion.	17	A	They are contradictory, with earlier studies promoting a slower shift change rate.
10	D	an illness caused by routine personal behaviors.	18	B	professionals being less aware of the danger they can pose.
11	A	effective interventions do not equal problem solving unless adopted routinely.	19	C	show that assessment of shift impact must focus on multiple factors.
12	C	Concurrent smoking and alcohol intake have a cumulative effect on bioavailability.	20	A	wariness that Li's results may be used to keep detrimental shift patterns.
13	A	profits and popular sentiment illogically drive ideas of good diet.	21	D	overall profits from longer shifts may be much less than assumed.
14	C	case studies.	22	C	Suggesting practicable measures to empower and support nurses

www.ingramcontent.com/pod-product-compliance
Lightning Source LLC
Chambersburg PA
CBHW081917090526
44590CB00019B/3390